£19.95

Drugs in S

D1355468

Eu

Edi

Jar

Pro:
Cer
Fac
Uni
Pre

ar

D

Dir
Ur
Ar

F

P

Groupe Pompidou
Pompidou Group

Radcliffe Publishing

Oxford • New York

Radcliffe Publishing Ltd
18 Marcham Road
Abingdon
Oxon OX14 1AA
United Kingdom

www.radcliffe-oxford.com
Electronic catalogue and worldwide online ordering facility.

British Library Cataloguing in Publication Data

A catalogue record for this book is available from the British Library.

ISBN-10 1 84619 093 2
ISBN-13 978 184619 093 3

Typeset by Anne Joshua & Associates, Oxford
Printed and bound by TJI Digital, Padstow, Cornwall

Contents

Foreword

Some time ago, after a day of listening to the presentations at a particularly uninspiring conference, a colleague remarked to me wearily and only half jokingly that things had gone far enough . . . no further research was necessary . . . we simply know everything that is worth knowing about drugs and those that use them. I admit that there has been the odd moment since when events have conspired to make me suspect that there may even be some wisdom in this proposition. It is therefore gratifying to be presented with the collection of papers that constitute *Drugs in Society – a European perspective* as it serves as a welcome antidote to such a cynical position. And in doing so it not only clearly illustrates the value of social research as a powerful tool for illuminating subjects that are too often overlooked in the discourse on the drug problem, but also reminds us why such a detailed vision is important.

This book contains a diverse and eclectic set of papers. In some texts this would be considered a weakness but here it merely serves to reflect the diverse and eclectic nature of drug use in Europe and, in doing so, makes for a rich reading experience. Furthermore, although the subject matter covered is broad, the papers are united in that they share a common perspective where drug use is not simply reduced to questions of dependence or compulsion, and where the principle concern is not only to audit consequences. Rather this book is about drug use as a dynamic social behaviour where understanding meaning and motivations, and culture and context, are as important as understanding the actions of chemicals on the brain or body. Some of the arguments are provocative and the reader may not agree with all the conclusions reached within these pages. What they will find is a set of papers that are stimulating to read, in part because they look at new things and in part because they look at old things differently.

Such an approach can only be welcomed as it serves to remind us of the diversity of the drugs issue itself. In Europe we have come a long way in developing a common approach to describing drug use based on standardising our data and developing comparable methods and measures. This approach does deliver benefits in allowing a simple common language for the European policy debate. It does, however, bring with it the risk that we over simplify and ignore the diversity of the European drug scene. Under the umbrella term 'drug use' we are talking about a complex set of behaviours – different drugs and different patterns of use, different motivations and different consequences, all influenced by time and place and the prevailing cultural and political context. It may be useful for many reasons to be able to describe general patterns of drug use in Europe but we forget at our peril the underlying reality of our subject matter.

The task of elaborating this reality, or perhaps even realities, has been one of the ongoing achievements of the European Society for Social Drug Research (ESSD), and this book owes it parentage to this group and its annual meetings. ESSD events are unlike many conferences as they demand, with threats if necessary, that you should not only attend but also participate. This, together with an emphasis on qualitative research and the regular presence of some of the more interesting and thought-provoking researchers working in Europe at the moment, has resulted in a series of conferences that stand apart for both their originality and vitality. In short, if you are feeling jaded and uninspired, and have forgotten why this topic ever interested you in the first place; if you simply want to read something provocative and different that reminds you of why the use of drugs is not only an important policy issue but also a fascinating area for social research – this book is for you – and these seem to me pretty good reasons for recommending a text.

Paul Griffiths
Scientific Co-ordinator, Situation Analysis
European Monitoring Centre for Drugs and Drug Addiction (EMCDDA)
Lisbon, Portugal
January 2007

About the editors

Professor Jane Fountain, PhD, has been working in the drug research field since 1988, and became a Professor of Substance Use Research in 2005. She is currently the lead on research at the Centre for Ethnicity and Health, University of Central Lancashire, UK. She previously worked as a researcher at the National Addiction Centre at the Institute of Psychiatry/Maudsley Hospital in London. She is a research consultant for several international organisations, her work has been widely published in academic journals, and she has edited several books.

Jane uses mainly qualitative research methods, most often to conduct research on drug use, drug treatment and other drug-related issues, particularly among so-called 'hidden' or 'hard-to-reach' populations and those vulnerable to problematic drug use.

Dirk J Korf, PhD, is associate professor in criminology at the Universities of Amsterdam and Utrecht. His main fields of research are patterns and trends in drug use and drug trafficking, drug policy, crime and crime prevention, and ethnic minorities. He has published many papers, reports and books on these issues. He is chair of the European Society for Social Drug Research (ESSD).

List of contributors

Sundari Anitha, PhD
Senior Lecturer (Research)
Centre for Ethnicity and Health, Faculty of Health
University of Central Lancashire
Preston
UK

Vibeke Asmussen, PhD
Associate Professor and Researcher
Centre for Alcohol and Drug Research
University of Aarhus
Aarhus
Denmark

Cas Barendregt, MA
Researcher
Instituut voor Onderzoek naar Leefwijzen and Verslaving
Rotterdam
The Netherlands

Brigitte Boon, PhD
Research Manager
Instituut voor Onderzoek naar Leefwijzen and Verslaving
Rotterdam
The Netherlands

Helle Vibeke Dahl, MA
Anthropologist
Centre for Alcohol and Drug Research
University of Aarhus
Aarhus
Denmark

Tom Decorte, PhD
Director of the Institute for Social Drug Research
Department of Penal Law and Criminology
Ghent University
Ghent
Belgium

Maria do Carmo Gomes, MSc
Researcher
Centro de Investigação e Estudos de Sociologia/Centre for Research and
Studies in Sociology (CIES-ISCTE)
Lisbon
Portugal

Axel Klein, PhD
Lecturer
Addictive Behaviour Group
Kent Institute of Medicine and Health Sciences
University of Kent
Canterbury
UK

Marjolein Muys, MA
Researcher
Institute for Social Drug Research (ISD)
University of Ghent
Ghent
Belgium

Alfred Springer, MD
University Professor
Ludwig–Boltzmann Institute for Addiction Research (LBISucht)
Vienna
Austria

Alfred Uhl, PhD
Senior Scientist
Ludwig–Boltzmann Institute for Addiction Research (LBISucht)
and Director
Alcohol Co-ordination and Information Centre (AKIS)
Federal Ministry of Health and Women
Anton Proksch Institute (API)
Vienna
Austria

Acknowledgements

This book's editors and contributors are all members of the European Society for Social Drug Research (ESSD), which was established in 1990. The principal aim of the ESSD is to promote social science approaches to drug research, with special reference to the situation in Europe. The editors thank Sundari Anitha, Vibeke Asmussen, Cas Barendregt, Brigitte Boon, Helle Vibeke Dahl, Tom Decorte, Maria do Carmo Gomes, Axel Klein, Marjolein Muys, Alfred Springer and Alfred Uhl for their diverse and interesting contributions to this aim, their painstaking responses to the editors' and peer reviewers' queries and comments, and their adherence to tight deadlines.

We gratefully thank the following individuals, who peer reviewed the authors' contributions, for their time and insightful comments: Nicole Crompton, Hermann Fahrenkrug, Ludwig Kraus, Bob McDonald, Aileen O'Gorman, Deborah Olszewski, Colm Power, Sharon Rödner, Alastair Roy, Sandrine Sleiman, Tim Thornton, Hylke Vervaeke and Marije Wouters.

We also thank the staff at Radcliffe Publishing, especially Gillian Nineham, for their efficiency and understanding.

Finally, the editors gratefully acknowledge the support of the Council of Europe Pompidou Group.

Introduction: the social meanings of drugs

Jane Fountain and Dirk J Korf

Drugs are more than chemical substances that influence individual human behaviour through their effect on the brain. Drug use is often a social activity that takes place in an environment with other users. In addition to a drug's pharmacological properties, the drug user's personality, attitudes, expectations and motivating factors, and especially the setting in which drug use occurs, have a great influence on both the user and their drug-using patterns.[1] Drugs may be used as a means of forgetting daily problems, such as poverty, unemployment, homelessness and mental ill health, but for other users they symbolise the 'sunny' side of life while partying and clubbing. The same substance can be used by different people for different reasons, and with different effects being experienced. Cocaine is a typical example. It is used as a 'street drug' by deviant and socially excluded groups, but is also popular among those who are socially well integrated. As in North America, the use of cocaine (in its powder or crack form) has become part of the drug-using repertoire of heroin addicts in many European countries, and among socially excluded groups its use is more prevalent than that of heroin.[2] However, the snorting of cocaine powder is also increasingly popular among young people in trendy urban nightlife settings. In these settings, cocaine has become a serious competitor with ecstasy,[3] the most popular party drug of the last decade in many European countries, including the new European Union (EU) member states.[4]

Drugs also have social meanings for non-users, and not only can the same drug – for example, cocaine – have different meanings at the same time, but also the social meaning of a particular drug can change drastically over time. Cannabis is probably the best example of this. Initially strongly stigmatised, the use of this drug was associated with individual pathology (such as cannabis psychosis and amotivational syndrome) in the early 1960s. However, it became redefined as a symbol of the youth protest subculture in the late 1960s and early

1970s. As cannabis use has increased further among the whole population in subsequent decades, sociologists today define it as 'normalised.'
This term may imply that the use of cannabis has become normal
behaviour among the general population, in particular amongst the
younger generation, but this is not a crucial element of the concept. At
the core of normalisation is the notion that the use of drugs – particularly
cannabis – has lost its exceptional status and has entered the realm of the
familiar and habitual.[5] Drug use among socially non-excluded people
(e.g. smoking cannabis or using cocaine powder or ecstasy on the club
scene) is now commonly described as 'recreational drug use.' Thus drug
use is no longer the exclusive preserve of a specific population, and is only
one of the many symbols of social distinction among young people,
together with a specific style of music, clothing, and so on.

Different ways of perceiving drugs

From general population data on social perceptions of drugs, drug users
and consequences of drug use in Portugal, Maria do Carmo Gomes
constructs a tripartite typology in Chapter 1. Almost half of the
Portuguese population perceives drugs as a health problem, and addiction as a curable illness. Members of this group are typically in their mid-
thirties to mid-forties, employed, oriented towards social stability in the
community, and have little experience of drugs and drug users. The other
half of the Portuguese population can be divided into two equally sized
subgroups. On the one hand, there are those who perceive drugs in terms
of lifestyle. For them, drug use can be a conscious choice and does not of
itself have negative social consequences. Members of this subgroup tend
to be young, often students or unemployed, more focused on the
individual, and close to (or part of) the social world of drug use. On
the other hand, there is a subgroup that perceives drugs as a social
problem. They identify drug users with specific youth cultures and/or
with social exclusion, criminality and stigmatisation. Members of this
subgroup are mostly older people, educated to a lower level, housewives
or retired, and with no experience of drugs or drug users. It is likely that
the distribution of the three types will not be identical across Europe, but
it appears that the typology itself is applicable to other countries, as there
are striking similarities with the results of an earlier study conducted in
urban areas in 11 European countries.[6]

At first sight, the chapter by do Carmo Gomes might seem to be in
conflict with the normalisation thesis. Only a quarter of the Portuguese
population aged 15 years or older perceive drugs as an expression of
lifestyle, but this was the dominant definition among young people – that
is, those who are most likely to be drug users or to be in contact with drug
users. Individuals in their late thirties and early forties tend to define drug

users as people with a health problem, and the older generation tends to define them in terms of deviance and crime. Indirectly, the Portuguese study has clearly illustrated the development of society's moral judgements of drug use, ranging from deviance (as perceived by today's senior citizens) to a health problem (as perceived by middle-aged adults), to an expression of lifestyle (as perceived by adolescents and young adults).

Dynamics of the cannabis market

Cannabis (known in its solid form as resin or hashish and in its herbal form as marijuana) is the most commonly used illegal drug across Europe. Within the EU around 62 million people have used cannabis at least once in their life, and approximately 20 million have used it during the past 12 months.[2] In a survey conducted among 15- to 16-year-old students in 35 European countries, a total of 21% reported that they had used the drug at least once in their life, with around 40% of respondents in the Czech Republic, France, Ireland and Switzerland having used it.[7] In the EU, between 11% and 44% of young people aged 15–34 years have tried cannabis at least once, with the highest rates in France (40%), the UK (43%) and Denmark (45%). Use within the last 12 months within the same age category ranges from 3% to 22%, and is highest in the UK and France (both 20%) and the Czech Republic (22%). Figures are higher in urban than in rural areas, but the difference has tended to decrease in recent years.

Cannabis appears to be relatively easily available. Although the prevalence of use peaks in late adolescence and early adulthood, over a third of 15- to 16-year-old students in Europe (and close to two-thirds of those in the UK and Ireland) report that hashish or marijuana is fairly or very easy to obtain.[7] Over 50% of students of this age say that they know of places where cannabis can easily be bought, such as discotheques and bars (27%), public places such as streets or parks (23%), a dealer's home (21%) or in and around school (16%). However, apart from coffee shops in the Netherlands, where the sale of small amounts of cannabis to consumers aged 18 years or over is tolerated under certain conditions, little is known about the structure of the cannabis market in Europe.

Until the late 1980s, the European cannabis market was largely supplied with imported hashish, in particular from Morocco. More recently, both commercial and non-commercial domestic cultivation of marijuana has increased with the advent of new growing techniques and crossbred varieties. Domestic cultivation of marijuana is now becoming increasingly professional, and criminal organisations have become involved. In Chapter 3, Tom Decorte describes and analyses this evolutionary process in Belgium and the Netherlands in terms of drug policy initiatives, arguing that it represents a process of 'import substitution', that it has also occurred in other European countries and in North America, and that it appears to be irreversible. Decorte believes that it is likely that the domestic production of hashish will be the next step in this market development.

The focus of the retail supply of cannabis has been for many years and still is on the Netherlands, but other European countries have an implicit history of tolerating the sale of hashish and marijuana to consumers. It is common for the police not to actively enforce laws against cannabis retail sales, particularly in urban areas (Switzerland is the only European country that intends to legalise the retail cannabis market). For example, for many years the sale of cannabis was tolerated in Denmark, including its sale in so-called 'hash clubs' (similar to the coffee shops in the Netherlands) in some cities, and on 'Pusher Street' in the Free City of Christiana in Copenhagen – probably the most well-known open cannabis market in Europe. However, since a change in government in 2001, Danish drug policy has taken a more repressive turn. In Chapter 2, Vibeke Asmussen discusses how this change was implemented in practice with regard to cannabis dealing. She describes the political agenda and the role of mass media with regard to the closing of Pusher Street, and her analysis clearly illustrates a classic problem that in criminology has become known as 'displacement.' The cannabis retail market in the Danish capital did not disappear when Pusher Street was closed, but merely resurfaced in other parts of the city.

Old drugs, new meanings

Many substances that are sold today on the illicit drugs market in Europe have been used for centuries. Typical examples include cannabis, opium and psilocybin (magic mushrooms). Some are relatively new, such as heroin, which was discovered in 1898 and was first used as a cough medicine and as a cure for morphine addiction. Ecstasy (methylenedioxy-methamphetamine (MDMA)) was patented in 1912, but medical experiments with the drug in the US army did not meet initial expectations, and it was not until the 1970s that psychotherapists experimented with the drug in order to revive memories and bring suppressed emotions to the surface.[8,9] Following these experiments, MDMA was perceived as an ideal way to relieve daily stress and to relate to personal and others' feelings.[10] From the mid-1980s onward, ecstasy and its 'loved-up' effects became a popular dance drug among clubbers and ravers.

Ephedra is a generic term for a number of extracts from ephedra-containing herbs that are known under their Chinese name, *Ma huang*. This drug contains ephedrine and pseudo-ephedrine, which act as stimulants in the same way as adrenaline. In the late 1990s, ephedra was introduced to the recreational drug market as a 'natural drug' or 'natural ecstasy.' In Chapter 4, Cas Barendregt and Brigitte Boon report a variety of reasons for using the drug according to a survey of ephedra users in the Netherlands, but these were largely gender-specific. Women's main reason for using ephedra was to lose weight, whereas men used it so that they could dance for longer. Barendregt and Boon also shed some light on the dynamics of the drug market. After ephedra was banned in the Netherlands in 2004, some of its users cut down their consumption, while others used alternative legal or illegal substances.

Khat is another 'old' drug that has been introduced to Europe in recent decades, predominantly within immigrant communities, especially Somalis. Today this stimulant is illegal in most European countries, the UK and the Netherlands being the exceptions. Although it is often maintained that khat is a part of Somali culture and tradition that should be allowed to continue in exile, Axel Klein argues in Chapter 5 that it was not widely used in Somalia until the 1970s, and he defines the rationale for khat-chewing among Somali immigrants in Europe as an 'invented tradition.' This has serious consequences for the social meaning of khat use. Not only are regulation mechanisms affected by migration, but also there is no cultural memory of socially acceptable use and harm reduction strategies. This locks a significant minority of persistent users into problematic khat-using patterns.

Minority ethnic groups and drug use

Immigrant communities may introduce new traditions in substance use to their host country, whether 'invented' (as in the case of khat, described above) or 'real' (as in the case of the anti-alcohol culture among many Muslims). Some immigrants may become important bridgeheads in the international drug trade because they have social and commercial ties to countries that produce drugs (e.g. heroin in Asia, cocaine in Latin America, hashish in Morocco). However, in the host country, immigrants may also begin to use drugs that, in their country of origin, were not available or were not part of their social world.

The opening of the borders between member states of the EU has strongly stimulated the mobility of its citizens, both for studying and for work. In contrast, access to Europe for immigrants from non-western countries has become much more difficult, and is largely restricted to political and war refugees. In Chapter 6, Marjolein Muys shows how drug use among asylum seekers and refugees can be understood as self-medication. Using a literature review, she argues that despite the existence of some protective factors, these groups are likely to self-medicate problems that originate from stress due to pre- and post-immigration resource loss (e.g. loss of cultural resources, family, social status and future perspectives). Muys builds a theoretical model around three issues. First, refugees lack sufficient coping resources to offset resource loss. Secondly, they have no control over their situation. Thirdly, their low self-esteem makes it likely that they will respond to stress in a passive–avoidant way.

In Chapter 7, taking a more sociological perspective, Sundari Anitha describes low self-esteem (along with shame, blame and secrecy) as one of the feelings that are captured by the concept of stigma – a negative attribute, trait or disorder that marks out or labels its bearer as different from 'normal' people and attracts social sanctions. Anitha argues that what is defined as normal behaviour varies according to the society in which it occurs. A fear of stigma may prevent problematic drug users from seeking help or hinder those in treatment from deriving lasting benefit from it. This chapter's focus is on the manifestations of stigma related to problematic drug use in prisons in England and Wales. Drawing on data collected from multiple sources, Anitha describes, analyses and interprets the experience of stigma in a prison culture. This is linked, for example, to the drugs used. Minority ethnic prisoners were found to be more likely to disclose crack cocaine use than the use of heroin, especially if they injected the latter. In the context of a male prison, any attempt to shed the stigma of drug use by accessing drug treatment services may also be fraught with the danger of losing social status, as it could be seen as flouting the dominant discourse of masculinity and invulnerability. This chapter is a strong plea for a culturally sensitive approach to drug service provision, both theoretically and practically. For example, Anitha reports that, for minority ethnic prisoners, the predominantly white composition of prison drug service teams is a major barrier to accessing their services (as it is for minority ethnic drug users in the community[11]). As an alternative, Anitha suggests the creation of ethnically diverse teams of culturally competent drug service providers, who can understand concerns about stigma and take proactive measures to improve drug service accessibility.

From morphine to methadone

Methadone has become the 'gold standard' in substitution treatment of heroin addicts, first in the USA and now in most European countries – over half a million heroin addicts are on methadone maintenance treatment in Europe. In Chapter 8, Alfred Springer describes how in Austria there is a diversified system that allows prescription of different opioid substances for maintenance purposes. Under this system, the drug used for substitution has shifted from methadone to slow-release morphine, as many clients prefer this medication. However, in 2004 a campaign that aimed to abolish slow-release morphine preparations in maintenance treatment stimulated a process that, according to Springer in his analysis of the discourse in Austria, will put an end to diversified medical treatment of opioid dependency. He critically discusses how morphine has become stigmatised – using the same arguments that were put forward against methadone in the past – and how this is threatening the Austrian system, which is in danger of returning to methadone as the only substitute medication in maintenance treatment.

In Chapter 9, Helle Vibeke Dahl studies the practice of methadone treatment in Denmark from a different angle. Her focus is on the perspective of those clients who play the 'methadone game' as a response to its prescription as a means of controlling and disciplining them. To these clients, methadone maintenance treatment represents far more than a medical substitution for heroin, as the aim of the game is to be in possession and control of the methadone itself.

Ethics in social drug research

Definitions of the drug problem change over time, and drug use is thus an ideal subject for social drug research. In recent years, the medical study of drug use has made significant progress, and much more is now known about how drugs work via the brain. In the field of treatment, the medically based ideology of evidence-based research results has gained much influence, and rather than viewing drug addiction as an expression of a deviant lifestyle or a means of dealing with socio-economic problems, drug addiction is defined as a brain disease.

Shifting perspectives, even shifts in paradigms, are prerequisites for the advance of science. However, a mono-dimensional shift in drug research towards the medical discipline carries serious risks. First, drug use is largely recreational and can only be fully understood within the social context of fashions and lifestyles. Treatment, even when primarily medical, is also a social event. This makes it difficult, if not sometimes impossible, to evaluate the interventions in the field of drug prevention and treatment along the classic lines of evidence-based methodologies. Secondly, drug use is a social problem. Even though some drug use has normalised among the younger generations, politicians and policy makers often have a different perspective and a strong impact on the research agenda. Implicitly or explicitly, these diverging perspectives are reflected in drug research, not only in the presentation of research findings, but even in apparently 'neutral' questionnaires administered in surveys. In the final chapter of this book, Alfred Uhl issues a provocative challenge to researchers to be more self-critical in order to promote the advancement of research. He argues that drug policy research is not value-free, that the role of a researcher is totally incompatible with the role of an advocate, and that the term 'evidence-based policy' is a contradiction in itself, meaning that evidence-based drug policy is a fallacy.

References

1 Zinberg NE. *Drug, Set and Setting: the basis for controlled intoxicant use.* New Haven, CT: Yale University Press; 1984.
2 European Monitoring Centre for Drugs and Drug Addiction (EMCDDA). *The State of the Drugs Problem in the European Union and Norway. Annual report 2005.* Lisbon: EMCDDA; 2005.
3 Nabben T, Quaak L, Korf DJ. *NL Trendwatch 2004–2005.* Amsterdam: Rozenberg Publishers; 2005.
4 Allaste AA. Changing circles. How recreational drug users become problem users. In: Decorte T, Korf DJ, editors. *European Studies on Drugs and Drug Policy.* Brussels: VUB Press; 2004.
5 Parker H, Aldridge J, Measham F *et al. Illegal Leisure: the normalisation of adolescent recreational drug use.* London: Routledge; 1998.
6 Korf DJ, Bless R, Nottelman N. Urban drug problems, policy makers and the general public. *Eur J Criminal Policy Res.* 1998; **6**: 337–56.
7 Hibell B, Andersson B, Bjarnasson T *et al. The ESPAD Report 2003. Alcohol and other drug use among students in 35 European countries.* Stockholm: Swedish Council for Information on Alcohol and Other Drugs (CAN) and the Pompidou Group at the Council of Europe; 2003.
8 Peroutka SJ. *Ecstasy: the clinical, pharmacological and neurotoxicological effects of the drug MDMA.* Boston, MA: Kluwer Academic Publishers; 1990.
9 Shulgin A, Shulgin A. *PiHKAL: a chemical love story.* Berkeley, CA: Transform Press; 1991.
10 Rosenbaum M, Morgan P, Beck J. Ethnographic notes on ecstasy use among professionals. *Int J Drug Policy.* 1989; **1**: 16–19.
11 Fountain J, Bashford J, Winters M *et al. Black and Minority Ethnic Communities in England: a review of the literature on drug use and related service provision.* London: National Treatment Agency for Substance Misuse; 2003.

Chapter 1

Perceptions of drugs and drug users in Portugal

Maria do Carmo Gomes

How are drugs and drug use perceived in Portugal? What opinions do the Portuguese hold about drug users, psychoactive substances, and the social consequences of involvement with drugs? Are there differences among the Portuguese population in their perceptions of drug use? These are some of the questions guiding the research that informs this chapter, for, as Becker has pointed out, drugs and the definitions associated with them are primarily an issue of moral judgement set within a specific social context.[1]

The main theoretical research aims were to gain an understanding of how opinions are constructed through social processes embedded in different social, legal and cultural contexts, and to understand the relationship of such opinions according to the characteristics of those who hold them. Thus the research had three analytical axes – structural, interactional and socio-cultural. The analytical model followed by the research seeks to identify precisely the different ways in which the Portuguese population perceive drugs. It also seeks to ascertain the factors that most strongly influence these opinions, taking into account the effect of differences in social origins, life conditions, cultural orientation, social values and interactions with drugs and drug users.[2] This approach to research on illicit drugs and drug addiction in Portugal has not been widely used. Preference has been given to drug users' viewpoints, in an attempt to understand their relationship with the substances used, drug-using careers, and their experiences of social exclusion and discrimination, interventions and legislation. Less prominence has been given to the way in which drugs, drug use and drug users are perceived by the general public. However, contemporary society and publicly and socially involved citizens increasingly demand that decisions on public policies such as those related to drug use and addiction be taken on the basis of solid and scientifically valid knowledge.

This chapter is divided into four parts. The first part describes the research methods. The aim of the second part is to place the Portuguese situation within the context of the European Union (EU) from the point of view of drug use and addiction, indicating its specific features and developments in recent years. The third part presents some of the results relating to Portuguese opinions on three fundamental dimensions – the drugs, the drug users and the social consequences of addiction. On the basis of multivariate analyses of the data, the fourth part presents and discusses the typology of different ways of perceiving drugs.

Methods

The research was conducted by a survey of a representative sample of the Portuguese population ($n = 1002$) aged 15 years or over and residing in mainland Portugal. The sample was stratified by age, gender, occupation, educational level and region. The questionnaire covered the different dimensions contained in the analytical model,[2] and was completed by face-to-face interviews during February 2005.

The structured questionnaire was designed on the basis of the three analytical axes – structural, interactional and socio-cultural – defined above. These axes allow the definition of the independent variables such as social class, age and gender, educational level (the structural axis), contact with drugs users and contexts of drug use (the interactional axis), and social values and cultural orientations (the socio-cultural axis). The dependent variables were those relating to the three ways of exploring perceptions of the drug phenomena, namely perceptions of drugs, drug users and the social consequences of drug use. All of the items on the questionnaire consisted of options from which respondents were asked to make a selection, and which were devised from theoretical and empirical results obtained from previous studies.

The data were analysed using SPSS/PC, and included univariate, bivariate and multivariate analyses. The bivariate analysis used the crosstabs command and Chi-square tests for statistical significance ($P < 0.05$). The multivariate analysis used the K-means cluster to identify a typology of ways of perceiving drugs using only the dependent variables and multiple correspondences (HOMALS) to turn the projection in a two-dimensional topological space.

The Portuguese context

In recent years, an increased effort has been made to collect statistical indicators on drug use and addiction in the EU. As a result of the work of the European Monitoring Centre for Drugs and Drug Addiction (EMCDDA),[3] relevant data on the national situation of some EU countries, including Portugal, are now available for the first time. These can be used to make international comparisons, particularly in a European context.

The EMCDDA's annual reports of the drug situation in each EU country[4] have demonstrated the relative seriousness of the drug problem in Portugal. There are high levels of HIV/AIDS infection among drug addicts, high levels of problematic drug use, particularly heroin, associated with increasing involvement in synthetic drug use,[5] and ever earlier initiation of young people into drug use.[6] Portugal also has one of the highest recorded levels of drug use in prisons in the EU, including widespread intravenous drug use[7] and a relatively high number of drug-related arrests and convictions (around 75% of those in custody are arrested for offences directly or indirectly related to drug use).

In addition, Portuguese society shows signs of lagging well behind other European countries at a structural level,[8] and statistical data have revealed a twin-track situation. On the one hand, the signs of advanced modernity and economic, social and cultural development, with regard to which Portuguese society is similar to the most developed countries in Europe, are plain to see. On the other hand, at the same time there are certain indicators that compare unfavourably with other European countries, including educational and literacy levels, poverty rates, rates of early school-leaving and educational failure, investment in research and development, penetration and use of information technology, rates of productivity and economic competitiveness.

Research on the relationship between social deprivation and drug dealing and use shows highly specific configurations in Portugal. In the conurbations of Lisbon and Oporto, there are concentrations of neighbourhoods in which drug dealing and use are prevalent.[9] At the same time, new drug-use zones have appeared, spreading in association with the concentration of young people in some regions where new universities were established in the last decade – for example, in the Vila Real district and in the Alentejo region.[10]

Portugal is a country on the road to modernity as far as drug addiction regulations and legislation are concerned. Under the policy of risk reduction and harm minimisation, the use of psychoactive substances was decriminalised in 2000. Other social action initiatives and programmes were also associated with this change in the law, such as the creation of Drug Addiction Dissuasion Committees and regulations on the work to be carried out by outreach teams among problematic drug users, particularly in neighbourhoods where there is a high level of drug use and dealing.

Nevertheless, compared with other EU countries, Portugal is in a serious position with regard to drug use and addiction. Accordingly, it is trying to counteract the negative trends in the indicators listed above with a set of political regulations and measures. These have, for the first time, moved the focus of interventions from essentially clinical, individual and treatment aspects to those of a more collective and sociological nature. However, since 2002, the tendency to move towards this mainstream European position has been called into question politically for several reasons. The external assessment conducted on the 1999–2003 National Anti-drug Campaign Strategy[11] clearly showed that a great deal remained to be done and that a number of the objectives had only been partially met. For example, increased synthetic drug use among young people is associated with individuals who have a long history of problematic use of drugs such as heroin, and there is also large-scale so-called 'recreational' use of substances such as cocaine and cannabis.[12]

Many questions about the drug problem in Portugal have yet to be answered, and the fact that the policies that have emerged in recent years have lacked continuity and integration has made it more difficult to attain the goals defined for the first stage of intervention in the drug addiction field. The National Strategy for 2005–2012 foresees a continuation of the work carried out to date, in terms of strengthening treatment structures and providing them close to the addict, but it places special emphasis on prevention, research, geographically coordinated and integrated action, and attention to new trends in drug use.

Intermittent policies on intervention combined with economic cycles of crisis and social difficulties have left Portuguese society with serious problems to confront at the beginning of the twenty-first century, and drug addiction is undoubtedly one of these problems. In a country where problematic drug use is closely related to social exclusion,[7] how do the Portuguese perceive illicit substances and their users, and what is the relevance of these perceptions to the drug policy debate and definitions?

Perceptions of drugs, drug users and the social consequences of drug use

When the Portuguese sample[2] was questioned about how they perceive the psychoactive substances commonly referred to as 'drugs', the responses most frequently selected were that there are 'several illicit substances that produce different effects and consequences in individuals' (90%) and that drugs are a 'serious social and criminal problem' (88%). The sample's agreement with the statement that 'illicit drugs are a part of every society and must be seen that way' was considerably less unanimous, with only 51% agreeing with it. For 73% of the sample, 'illicit drugs production is an economic life resource for many poor populations around the world', although somewhat fewer (67%) supported the idea that 'if the financial interests related to drug trafficking end, drugs will become legal' (67%). These results clearly demonstrate the tendency to perceive drugs as a problem with serious consequences for society, rather than as an intrinsic element of every society.

With regard to illicit drug users, the data reveal the predominance of the notion of chemical addiction to a substance (87%). In total, 41% of the sample thought that all drug users are addicts, while 46% thought that many of them are. Addiction is therefore one of the characteristics of drug use that was prevalent in the opinions of the sample. The second most popular opinion (accounting for 86% of the sample) was that drug users are ill. Over half of the respondents (53%) agreed that all drug users are ill and should be treated clinically to enable them to recover, and 33% considered that many users are ill.

The third most popular opinion, with which 85% of the sample agreed, is that drug users 'are youngsters who do not think of the consequences of their actions for their future.' In total, 49% of the sample agreed that this applies to many drug users, while 36% considered that it applied to all of them. Over three-quarters of the sample (78%) considered that users of illicit drugs are 'people who live in situations of social exclusion.' Only 24% of the sample associated this characteristic with all users of illicit drugs, although over half (55%) believed that many drug users are in this situation.

A smaller proportion of respondents associated the following characteristics with illicit drug users: 'they are just like other people but have chosen a different lifestyle' (53%, with 17.5% thinking that all drug users have chosen a different lifestyle); 'they are criminals and must be judged and punished as such' (50%, with 19% thinking that all drug users are criminals); and they are individuals who 'consciously choose to use drugs and weigh up their advantages and disadvantages' (30%, with 9% thinking that all drug users have made this choice).

These results clearly indicate that there is no unanimous opinion in Portuguese society on the characteristics of illicit drug users. One trend is generally conservative and views drug users as criminals and deviants from the social norm. Another trend is more liberal, viewing drug users as equal to others, but as having chosen a different lifestyle. Finally, there are those who perceive drug users as having a health problem connected to addiction.

With regard to the social consequences of drug addiction (*see* Figure 1.1), the sample almost unanimously agreed that 'illicit drug use is always serious or very serious for drug users' health.' Only 4% disagreed with this statement, but 70% disagreed with the statement that 'illicit drug users have easier and happier lives than most people', and 48% disagreed with the statement that drug users 'can have as successful school careers and professional careers as anybody else.'

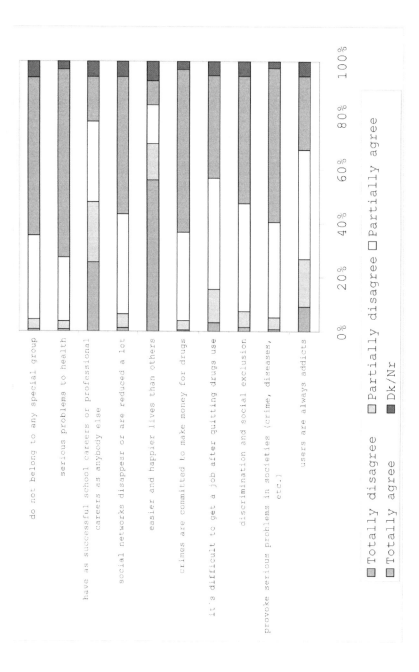

Figure 1.1: Perceptions of social consequences of drug use and abuse.

With regard to the stigma-related consequences of drug use, 27% of the sample disagreed with the statement that 'drug users are always seen as addicts even if they have stopped using drugs for a long period', and 16% disagreed with the statement that 'for users it is difficult to find a job after a treatment or recovery period.' However, only 7.5% disagreed with the statement that 'discrimination and social exclusion are inevitable consequences of illicit drug addiction.'

In some cases, when opinions were given on abstract categorisations such as social exclusion, discrimination was more strongly associated with drug use and addiction than when opinions were given on day-to-day situations such as finding a job. Paradoxically, 88% of the sample associated the disappearance of social networks with drug use, 92% agreed with the statement that 'illicit drug users cause a lot of problems and disquiet in society', and around 90% agreed that illicit drug users come from all social classes, and that crimes are committed in order to fund drug use. However, different distributions appear when these data are analysed according to independent variables such as social characteristics, closeness to drug contexts, and social and cultural attitudes. This analysis identified four trends, derived from bivariate analysis through variables that were statistically significant by Chi-square testing.

The first trend is that people with higher educational and occupational qualifications, adults, and those who are employed are more likely to perceive drug use as an individual problem of chemical addiction and to view drug users as people who are ill. This group also believes most strongly in the treatment and reversibility of drug addiction, and in recovery from it. The second trend indicates a more conservative and repressive outlook that is especially widespread among those with the lowest educational and occupational qualifications, the unemployed (including housewives and pensioners) and older people. It is based on a more discriminatory outlook that maintains with greater vigour that drug addiction is permanent or long-term. The third trend clearly shows that the closer the Portuguese are to illicit drug users and contexts of illicit drug use, the more liberal and permissive their perception of drug addiction tends to be. These results are consistent with the findings of a research project that was conducted in 11 European countries in the late 1990s.[13] The fourth trend, based on social and cultural attitudes, is that individuals with a more self-centred individualistic perspective on life, and whose values are more strongly associated with risk and adventure, are less likely to have a repressive or conservative opinion of drug use and drug users.

Ways of perceiving drugs in Portugal

Having presented the main trends in Portuguese opinion on drugs, drug users and the social consequences of drug use, in this section I shall

Table 1.1: Typology of ways of perceiving drugs in Portugal*

Statement	Health problem	Social problem	Lifestyle	Total
Social perceptions of drugs (0 = no; 1 = yes)				
There are several illicit substances considered as drugs that produce different effects and consequences in individuals	0.98	0.98	0.91	0.96
Illicit drugs production is an economic life resource for many poor populations around the world	0.76	0.84	0.87	0.81
Illicit drugs are a part of every society and must be seen that way	0.45	0.62	0.75	0.58
If financial interests related to drug trafficking end, drugs will become legal	0.75	0.80	0.80	0.78
Illicit drugs are a serious social and criminal problem and must be eliminated/eradicated from society	0.95	0.98	0.84	0.93
Social perceptions of drug users (1 = all of them; 4 = none of them)				
Illicit drug users are people who live with a strong addiction to chemical substances	3.37	3.64	3.08	3.36
Illicit drug users are just like other people, but have just chosen a different lifestyle	2.51	2.68	2.89	2.66
Illicit drug users are criminals and must be judged and punished as such	2.16	3.63	2.27	2.57
Illicit drug users are ill and must be treated clinically to recover from their addiction	3.54	3.40	3.26	3.42
Illicit drug users are youngsters who do not think of the consequences of their actions for their future	3.27	3.53	2.99	3.26
Illicit drug users consciously choose to use drugs, and weigh up their advantages and disadvantages	1.49	2.42	2.68	2.06
Illicit drug users are people who live in situations of social exclusion	2.98	3.39	2.92	3.07
Social perceptions of consequences of drug use (1 = totally agree; 4 = totally disagree)				
Illicit drug users are always drug addicts even if they can stop using drugs for a long period	2.61	3.66	2.68	2.90
Illicit drug users cause a lot of problems and disquiet in society, such as increased crime, spread of diseases, etc.	3.53	3.85	3.13	3.50
Discrimination and social exclusion are inevitable consequences of illicit drugs addiction	3.45	3.71	3.03	3.40

Table 1.1 (*cont.*)

Statement	Health problem	Social problem	Lifestyle	Total
For illicit drug users it is difficult to get a job after a period of treatment or recovery connected with drug addiction	3.17	3.68	2.77	3.19
The majority of drug users' crimes are committed in order to obtain money to maintain consumption patterns	3.69	3.82	3.17	3.58
Illicit drug users have easier and happier lives than most people	1.14	2.25	**2.48**	1.80
After drug addiction begins, drug users' social networks and sociability with family, friends and colleagues tend to diminish or disappear	3.51	3.75	3.09	3.45
Illicit drug users can have as successful school careers and/or professional careers as anybody else	2.29	2.25	**3.10**	2.50
The consequences of illicit drug use are always serious or very serious for drug users' health	**3.76**	3.93	3.20	3.65
Illicit drug users are people of all ages, and men and women from all social classes and regions, not belonging to any special group	3.69	**3.68**	3.33	3.59

* The K-means clusters method was used. The three ways of perceiving drugs presented here are the result of an earlier phase of data analysis, with the interpretation of solutions for 2, 4, 5 and 6 groups. This seemed the most appropriate solution from the viewpoint both of statistical requirements and of the sociological interpretability of the profiles identified. The values in bold represent the highest average obtained in each cluster for each variable.

attempt to examine in more depth the different ways in which this phenomenon is perceived, and how these ways are characterised. Using K-means cluster analysis,[14] three ways in which this phenomenon is perceived can be clearly identified (*see* Table 1.1), namely drugs as a health problem, as a social problem and as a lifestyle choice.

The variables that reflect drug use as a curable illness appear in association with the health problem cluster. This is the most popular perception of the Portuguese population sample (46%). The second most popular perception, of drugs as a lifestyle choice, brings together the views that drug use can be a conscious choice or an alternative way of living, that the production and distribution of illicit drugs are means of economic survival for certain populations, and that drug use has limited negative social consequences. Those who position themselves in this cluster represent 27.5% of the sample. The third cluster brings together

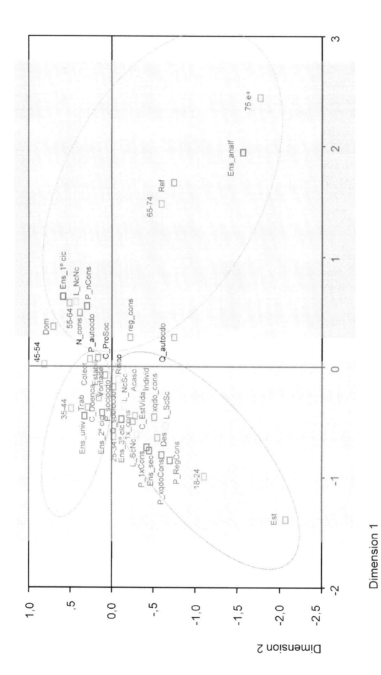

Figure 1.2: Ways of perceiving drugs in Portugal: topological space.

the views (of 26% of the sample) that identify drug use as a social problem. These include, for example, discrimination and social exclusion, crime, difficulties with social and professional integration, stigmatisation, and drug use as a specific characteristic of young people's behaviour.[15]

To complement these results, a multiple correspondence analysis (HOMALS) was employed, which allows the portrayal of the distribution of the association of the variables in a topological space (*see* Figure 1.2).

It clearly emerges from an analysis of dimension 1 (the vertical line that indicates the extent to which respondents have a relationship with drug-using contexts) that there is a difference between the Portuguese who have no such relationship (the right-hand side of the vertical axis), and those who do, and who include some drug users (the left-hand side of the vertical axis). Thus those respondents who view drugs as a social problem are associated with the right-hand side of Figure 1.2, and those who view drugs as a lifestyle or health problem are associated with the left-hand side.

An analysis of dimension 2 (the horizontal line that defines differences among the sample's social characteristics) provides additional information that distinguishes three groups within the topological space. They are identifiable by the dotted ellipses, confirming the three ways of perceiving drugs and the characteristics associated with each of these. On the right-hand side of the vertical axis are those who perceive drugs as a social problem, an opinion that is associated with individuals who are older (over 55 years of age), the unemployed (including housewives and pensioners), those with little education, and those who have no contact with drug-using contexts. Thus the analysis that was performed for dimension 1 is largely confirmed.

The left-hand side of Figure 1.2 is divided into two subgroups. One is the group of Portuguese people associated with the health problem cluster, namely those in employment, aged between 35 and 44 years and educated to a higher level. Their social and cultural orientations are stability and individual responsibility within a socially focused perspective on life, and they have little contact with drugs and drug users. The other subgroup consists of individuals associated with the lifestyle cluster, with social characteristics that are also pronounced. They are younger, they are unemployed or students, their social and cultural orientations are more self-centred and directed towards risk, adventure and individualism, and they are closely associated with drug-using contexts.

The identification of these three groups, structured in this way in the topological space of Portuguese society, constitutes an unquestionable contribution to our knowledge of the way in which populations perceive the phenomenon of drug use.

Conclusion

The aim of the research described in this chapter was to explore a dimension that has hitherto been little addressed in studies on illicit drug use and addiction. Some significant results have been obtained in terms of explaining how the Portuguese population's opinions of drug users and the uses of drugs are structured, and their relationship with other social dimensions. The most significant result is the identification, through the multidimensional analysis, of three different ways of perceiving drugs – as a health problem, as a social problem and as a lifestyle choice. This final result of a rather complex set of statistical operations has shown how independent and dependent variables interact.

In addition to the empirical importance of these results, it is useful to discuss why the opinions of the population in Portugal about the drugs phenomenon have such a configuration and structure and why, in countries with different social, legal and cultural contexts, the results may be different. The relationships between contexts and opinions are mediated by complex processes that lend themselves to in-depth analysis. Some of the independent variables used in this quantitative approach (such as proximity to the drugs world) could be very important in this process. Socio-cultural orientations, such as values and perspectives on life, could also be significant in influencing opinions on drug issues. However, it is important to investigate the links between a country's drug policies and its population's opinions, and this could be achieved by comparative approaches. Drug policy makers should consider the results of scientific research, such as the findings of the study reported here, but it could be more important to understand the influence of policy on the opinions of the general population. In the case of the Portuguese population, the relationship between health policy and the fact that almost half of the sample in this study perceived drugs as a health problem merits further investigation. The challenge to policy makers is whether they are prepared to move drug policy in the direction of greater liberalisation, greater medical assistance or greater repression, in accordance with what the population thinks about the issue.

References

1 Becker HS. Les drogues: que sont-elles? [Drugs: what are they?] In: Becker HS, editor. *Qu'est-ce qu'une Drogue? [What is a Drug?]* Anglet: Atlantica; 2001.
2 Gomes MC. *Modos de Percepção e Relação com os Consumos de Drogas em Portugal: esboços para a definição de um modelo [Ways of Perceiving and Ways of Relating with Drugs in Portugal: headlines for an analytical model].* Lisbon: Programa de Doutoramento em Sociologia do ISCTE (PhD paper); 2005.
3 For more information, see www.emcdda.eu.int/index.cfm (accessed 15 December 2005).

4 Based on EMCDDA's annual reports on drugs in the EU; www.emcdda.eu.int (accessed 15 December 2005).

5 Based on 2003 ESPAD report; www.drogas.pt/media/relatorios/investigacao/espad_2003_eu/ESPAD_cover.pdf (accessed 15 December 2005).

6 Based on EMCDDA's annual reports and the Portuguese Institute of Drugs (IDT) reports; www.emcdda.eu.int and www.drogas.pt (accessed 15 December 2005); Henriques S. *O Universo do Ecstasy. Contributos para uma análise dos consumidores e ambientes [The Ecstasy's Universe. An analysis of users and contexts]*. Azeitão: Autonomia; 2003.

7 Torres AC, Gomes MC. *Drogas e Prisões em Portugal [Drugs and Prisons in Portugal]*. Lisbon: IPDT/Ministério da Saúde; 2002; Torres AC, Gomes MC. *Drugs and Prisons in Portugal. Synopsis and technical appendix*. Lisbon: CES-ISCTE (summary report); 2002; Torres AC, Gomes MC. Drogas e prisões: relações próximas [Drugs and prisons: close relationships]. *Toxicodependências*. 2005; **11**: 23–40.

8 Viegas JML, Costa AF, editors. *Crossroads to Modernity. Contemporary Portuguese society*. Oeiras: Celta Editora; 2000; Costa AF, Mauritti R, Martins SC *et al.* Social classes in Europe. *Portug J Soc Sci*. 2002; **1**: 5–39; Cardoso G, Costa AF, Conceição CP *et al. A Sociedade em Rede em Portugal [The Social Network in Portugal]*. Oporto: Campo das Letras; 2005.

9 Chaves M. *Casal Ventoso: da Gandaia ao Narcotráfico [Casal Ventoso: an ethnographic approach]*. Viseu: Imprensa de Ciências Sociais, Colecção Estudos e Investigações, Centro de Investigações Sociais; 1999; Cunha MI. *Entre o Bairro e a Prisão: tráfico e trajectos [Between the Neighborhood and the Prison: narcotraffic and pathways]*. Oporto: Fim de Século Edições; 2002; Fernandes L. *O Sítio das Drogas [The Drugs Location]*. Lisbon: Editorial Notícias, Colecção Comportamentos; 1998.

10 Based on the annual reports of the Portuguese Institute of Drugs (IDT); www.drogas.pt (accessed 15 December 2005).

11 Instituto Nacional de Administração. *Avaliação Externa da ENLCD 1999–2004 [External Evaluation of the National Strategy against Drugs 1999–2004]*. Lisbon: Portuguese Institute of Drugs (IDT); 2005.

12 Instituto da Droga e da Toxicodependencia (IDT). *National Report on Drug Situation in Portugal*. Lisbon: Portuguese Institute of Drugs (IDT); 2005.

13 Korf DJ, Bless R, Nottelman N. Urban drug problems, policy makers and the general public. *Eur J Criminal Policy Res*. 1998; **6**: 337–56.

14 Similar to the methodology followed by Costa AF, Ávila P, Mateus S. *Públicos da Ciência [The Public Face of Science]*. Lisbon: Gradiva; 2002.

15 Pais JM. *Culturas Juvenis [Youth Cultures]*. Lisbon: Imprensa Nacional Casa da Moeda; 1993; Pais JM. *Jovens 'Arrumadores de Carros': a sobrevivência nas teias da toxicodependência [Young Car Watchers: surviving drug addiction]*. Lisbon: ICS; 2001; Pais JM. *Ganchos, Tachos e Biscates. Jovens, Trabalho e Futuro [Young People, their Work and Future]*. Oporto: Ambar, Colecção Trajectórias; 2001.

Chapter 2

Danish cannabis policy in practice: the closing of 'Pusher Street' and the cannabis market in Copenhagen

Vibeke Asmussen

During the last three or four years, Danish drug policy has been reversed from liberal to more repressive, especially in 2003, when the Danish liberal–conservative government that had been in office since 2001 launched their official policy on drugs, *The Fight Against Drugs: action plan against drug misuse*.[1] This action plan emphasised a more repressive drug policy in which priority was given to law enforcement, although an expansion of treatment facilities and prevention initiatives was also planned. The overall aim was to tighten the laws on drug dealing and drug use and to increase the penalties for these offences. The plan explicitly stated that the policy was to take a zero tolerance approach towards any kind of drug dealing.

The fact that the liberal–conservative wing of the Danish parliament holds this attitude is not new. Storgaard[2] argues that the different drug control policies of this wing (which do not differentiate between users and dealers, or between 'hard' and 'soft' drugs) and the centre-left (which do) have been a battlefield in Danish drug policy for the past 30 years. The centre-left wing, headed by the Social Democratic Party, dominated Danish drug policy until 2001, when the present liberal–conservative government came into office. Although the Social Democratic Party did tighten some aspects of their drug policy, whether they would have continued to do so to the extent that the liberal–conservatives subsequently did is a matter for speculation.

One aspect of the present government's more repressive drug policy was to crack down on cannabis dealing as well as cannabis use. The focus of this chapter is the closing of 'Pusher Street', one of the most well-known places for buying cannabis in Copenhagen, the capital of Denmark. Pusher Street, named by the government as Northern Europe's largest open cannabis market, has been situated in the Free City of Christiania from the mid-1970s. In 2003, it consisted of about 40 decorated stalls where different kinds of cannabis were sold. Over the years, there have been police actions, raids and arrests of dealers in Pusher Street,[3–5] but there had never been a political decision or an organised operation to close it. However, in March 2004 the stalls were removed in a massive police action, and 50 cannabis dealers and 'security guards' (lookouts to warn the dealers of approaching police) were arrested.[6]

Studies of cannabis policy[7,8] show that repressive policies do not have an effect on the consumption of cannabis or, it can be deduced from this, on its supply. When investigating the effect of police actions and raids, the question of where and how cannabis dealing emerges again is raised, although research into locations, the size of the market, personnel and turnover is hampered, as it is with any criminal activity, by the hidden nature of the activity.[9] In Copenhagen, cannabis was sold from Pusher Street, from 'hash clubs' (which can be compared to Dutch coffee shops where cannabis is sold and consumed, but are totally illegal in Denmark[10]), in the street, from cars and homes, and via the telephone and the Internet.

This chapter outlines the drug-related legal changes that have recently been made in Denmark, and describes how their implementation supports the government's more repressive drug policy. Pusher Street is then contextualised and a short history of Christiania is provided, demonstrating how both have become thorns in the government's side. The chapter continues with an analysis of how Pusher Street was closed and kept closed, how cannabis dealing was then dispersed across Copenhagen, and how two methods of dealing (hash clubs and street dealing) in particular were brought to public attention by the newspapers. The chapter ends with a discussion of why some parts of the dispersed cannabis market were brought to public attention and others were not.

Newspapers and claim makers

The description and analysis of the situation is based on newspaper articles from three national Danish newspapers from March 2004 to April 2005,[11] the year after Pusher Street was closed. The political perspective of these newspapers can be broadly characterised as liberal–conservative (*Jyllands-Posten*), conservative (*Berlingske Tidende*) and centre-left (*Politiken*). The papers differed in the amount of coverage they gave to Pusher Street and the cannabis market in Copenhagen. *Jyllands-Posten* printed 42 articles in the period (23 articles about the closing of Pusher Street and how it was kept closed, and 19 articles about the cannabis market in Copenhagen). *Berlingske Tidende* printed 25 articles (15 articles about the closing of Pusher Street and aftermath, eight about the cannabis market in Copenhagen, and two on other cannabis-related issues). *Politiken* printed 24 articles (seven on the closing of Pusher Street and the aftermath, and 17 articles on the cannabis market in Copenhagen). *Jyllands-Posten* in particular followed the efforts by the police to keep cannabis dealing out of Pusher Street, and *Berlingske Tidende* covered this aspect, too, but less extensively. *Politiken* covered the dispersed cannabis market in more detail than the other two papers.

The papers differed in their sources of information, and therefore differed in the groups to whom they gave a voice as a claim maker.[12] The claim makers used can be categorised as the police, politicians, cannabis users, cannabis dealers, citizens (neighbours, parents, and inhabitants of Christiania) and professionals (researchers, social workers and lawyers). Some articles used more than one category of claim maker, while others did not use any. It is clear from the articles based on quotes from claim makers (*see* Table 2.1) that the police were used most often by all three newspapers, and that *Politiken* used a wider variety of claim makers than the other two papers.

The individual categories of claim maker did not always speak with a common voice, apart from the police, who always presented a particular perspective in all three newspapers, namely that the police actions against cannabis dealing were necessary, that the actions on Pusher Street were a success, and that police intervention is the only way to

Table 2.1: Quotes on cannabis and the cannabis market from claim makers in the three Danish newspapers during the period March 2004 to April 2005

Claim maker	Jyllands-Posten	Berlingske Tidende	Politiken
Police	34	16	11
Politicians	1	1	2
Cannabis users	3	–	4
Cannabis dealers	–	1	4
Citizens	10	1	3
Professionals	2	1	4
Total number of articles using claim makers	39	18	17
Total numbers of articles using two or more categories of claim maker	7	2	9
Total number of published articles on the cannabis market	42	25	24

combat drug crime. All of the categories of claim makers stated that the cannabis market is difficult to remove permanently, but held different opinions as to whether a repressive drug policy is constructive or not. Professionals, cannabis dealers and citizens were often used as claim makers to represent different perceptions and experiences from those of the police. The police were used particularly often when the papers reported on the situation in Pusher Street, while other claim makers were more often used when the relocated cannabis market was discussed.

In reporting on the situation, the three newspapers presented not only the claim makers' points of view, but also their own, according to their political agenda and when pursuing a 'good story.' The newspapers' viewpoints on cannabis policy were expressed in their editorials, which during March 2004 all supported the closing of Pusher Street and the new drug policy. A year later, the editorials differed, and although they all considered that the cannabis market could not be removed completely, they argued this from different angles. *Jyllands-Posten* supported the police actions, and argued that Pusher Street should have been closed many years ago. *Berlingske Tidende* emphasised that the police should do everything they can to obstruct the cannabis market. *Politiken*, on the other hand, interpreted the police action not only against Pusher Street, but also against the cannabis market in general in Copenhagen, as a complete fiasco, since no real change in cannabis distribution in Copenhagen had occurred following the police actions. However, none of the newspapers argued for the legalisation of cannabis. The 'good story' that the newspapers pursued was, for example, exposing police failure to control the cannabis market, or basing reports on the anxiety – or panic – related to drugs that has made them society's 'Enemy Number One',[13] especially in relation to young people and the risk of them becoming addicts. The point here is that the attention that the cannabis market in Copenhagen received in the three newspapers after the closing of Pusher Street is related to specific views and perceptions of drugs in general and drug policy in particular. The analysis of the cannabis market presented here is therefore only a partial analysis, as it focuses on the aspects that the newspapers brought to public attention.

Legal changes during the period 2001–2005

The more repressive approach in Danish drug policy has been implemented by the tightening of several legal issues over the past few years. The first of these, which came in 2001, was the Law Prohibiting Visitors to Designated Places, popularly referred to as the Hash Club Law.[14] This law was initiated in response to a media debate – with a tendency towards moral panic – concerning young people and their use of hash clubs,[10] and was implemented to enable the police to close them down, which had been impossible under the previous drug laws. The law was reinterpreted by the new government in 2005 so as to make it even easier to implement. The number of offences that had to have been committed by a hash club for it to be closed down (such as the presence of cannabis, or people using it, on the premises) was reduced from 10 to 15 offences to three to five.

In 2004, two areas of the Law on Euphoria-Inducing Substances were revised.[15] First, possession of cannabis for personal use is now punishable with a minimum of a fine. Before the revision, possession of up to 10 grams of cannabis for personal use would not result in prosecution. Since the revision it has been illegal to possess any amount of any illegal drug, and the former differentiation between users (who were not criminalised) and dealers (who were) has been eliminated. Secondly, the penalties for selling drugs to children and young people under the age of 18 years were increased from a fine to a prison term. Other penalties for drug-related crimes were also increased when the Prison Law was amended in 2004.[16] The maximum prison sentence for drug possession offences was raised from 6 to 10 years, and for trafficking and dealing it was raised from 10 to 16 years (or up to 24 years for very large amounts).[2] At the same time, the opposition parties (including the Social Democratic Party) proposed the legalisation of cannabis, the provision of safe injection rooms, and trials of heroin prescribing for heroin users in treatment. All of these proposals were outvoted in parliament.[17]

The tightening of the drug laws means that a control policy that differs between users and dealers and between 'soft' and 'hard' drugs is no longer at the heart of Danish drug policy, and it is a radical change that the use of cannabis is now a crime. Given that cannabis is the most widely used illegal drug in Denmark (as elsewhere), a large number of people have been criminalised by these legal changes.[2] In *The Fight Against Drugs: action plan against drug misuse*,[1] one of the government's arguments for enhancing law enforcement and increasing penalties for drug offences is to prevent drug use among young people, and the legal changes reflect this. Young people are protected by the revision, since the penalty for dealing drugs to young people has been raised from a fine to a prison term. However, cannabis users – many of whom are young people[18–20] – are now criminalised for the possession of cannabis for personal use.

Christiania and Pusher Street

Christiania was founded in 1971, when the government closed barracks located on around 34 hectares of land, and the old military area was almost immediately occupied by young squatters. Soon more than several hundred young people had begun to establish their vision of an 'alternative' society based on values such as autonomy, community, freedom, love and sustainability. Many of the first squatters were hippies, and they were anti-authoritarian and anti-bourgeois. The occupation must be seen as a child of its time and in relation to the youth revolt in the 1960s, and the new movements such as the peace movement, the sexual revolution and the women's liberation movement.[5] The Free City of Christiania has become the second largest tourist attraction in Copenhagen after Tivoli, and today has about 600 inhabitants and contains more than 80 different kinds of businesses, art studios, restaurants, bars and cafés.[21,22] Many cultural events are arranged in Christiania, including rock concerts, theatre performances and art exhibitions.

From the inception of Christiania, cannabis use was part of life there, as it was part of the youth revolt in general in the 1960s and 1970s. Christiania thus became synonymous with cannabis and arguments about legalising the drug. For example, from 1997 to 2001, yearly 'Hearings about hash, hemp and culture' were arranged in Christiania to discuss the current cannabis policy and situation in Denmark, with different experts being invited to participate. The conclusions of the debates were that legalisation of cannabis was the only constructive way to solve the dilemmas with regard to cannabis.[22] The relationship between cannabis dealing and Christiania has been debated intensely in Parliament over the years, and has resulted in regular police interventions and raids in Pusher Street and the rest of Christiania.[3–5,23]

Many Members of Parliament have strongly objected to the existence of Christiania, but it has survived through changes of government, and different plans and strategies have been put forward for its development. In 1991, an agreement was made that the government accepted Christiania but did not legalise it. This agreement was renegotiated every year, and in 1998 it was signed for a five-year period. However, in 2003 the present liberal–conservative government did not renew the agreement, and instead it initiated plans to 'legalise' Christiania. A parliamentary committee has been working on this issue, and reported on it in 2004.[24] Christiania has also produced a plan for its future,[22] as has Copenhagen's building and housing administration.[25] In its 'legalisation' plans, the present government wants to address not only the illegal activities in Christiania (the illegal use and occupation of military property, cannabis dealing and the cannabis market) but also governance, by switching Christiania's communal management of housing to the regulations for public and private housing that govern the rest of Denmark (Christiania is well placed in the centre of Copenhagen, and in recent years the surrounding areas have developed into an attractive neighbourhood with expensive housing).

The government's plans to legalise Christiania have significant implications for Christiania's basis of governance, which has always been a participatory democracy. Every inhabitant of Christiania can participate in any forum or meeting, including the Communal Meeting, which is Christiania's supreme authority, and decisions are only taken when consensus has been reached. The structure of government has developed during the past 35 years, but Christiania is now divided into 14 areas, each with 10 to 80 inhabitants and their own autonomous forum. This means that, for example, rules for the assignment of houses differ according to each area. Housing in Christiania consists of the old military buildings and newly built houses. Many of the new houses are built in alternative styles, using unconventional material, painted in bright colours, and built according to ideas of sustainable development for society. The inhabitants cannot own the house where they live, because it is on military property. If they move away, the area forum decides who will take over the house.[22] This collective governing of housing will disappear with the government's plans to legalise the area. Instead, other forms of ownership or administration of ownership are planned, such as selling the area at its market price or allowing organisations based on representative democracy and elected boards to administer it. Therefore Christiania as an alternative society with an alternative form of governing will disappear.

Implementation of the zero tolerance policy

A historical date in Danish drug policy is 16 March 2004. On this date, the police action to close down Pusher Street began at 5 a.m. Bulldozers and several hundred armed police officers entered Christiania and removed all the stalls from which cannabis was sold. Simultaneously, over 50 cannabis dealers and security guards were arrested in Christiania and elsewhere in Copenhagen and remanded in custody.[6] Within a few hours, a cannabis market that had existed for over 30 years was closed. The police action was peaceful in the sense that neither the cannabis dealers nor the inhabitants of Christiania made any attempts to resist the action.

The police action was thoroughly planned. A press release was used by the three newspapers that were analysed for this study, and this made it clear that Pusher Street had been under police surveillance for the previous six months, that radio communication and telephone calls had been tapped, that undercover police officers had bought cannabis there (the use of undercover police officers in Denmark is exceptional and requires a court's permission), and that Swedish and Norwegian police officers had joined the Danish police for the operation. The press release gave these detailed accounts of the police work in order to expose the fact that the cannabis market in Pusher Street was well organised.

All three newspapers supported the closure of Pusher Street. They all covered the closure and the immediate aftermath in detail for up to two weeks, and used the police as the major claim makers. During this period, only one article in each newspaper used other claim makers. *Jyllands-Posten* interviewed a cannabis user and regular customer in Pusher Street on where to buy cannabis now that Pusher Street was closed, *Berlingske Tidende* quoted a representative from Christiania about his view of the police action, and *Politiken* reported on the distribution of cannabis in Christiania immediately after the police action, using investigative reporting. The newspapers all reported the police action as a success and a necessary step, but also began to speculate about where the cannabis market would resurface, suggesting that it would be in hash clubs and via telephone-based delivery services.

During the following year, the level of police presence in Christiania varied from armed police constantly patrolling Christiania and Pusher Street, to patrols a few times a day, to random patrols. Constant patrolling was reinstated for a period if there had been clashes between the police and cannabis dealers, cannabis users and/or inhabitants of Christiania. For example, between December 2004 and June 2005, several of those arrested in the police raids on Pusher Street in March 2004 were released,[6] and the papers described clashes between them and the dealers who had taken over the cannabis market. In April 2005, it was reported that a young man was shot in Christiania and several others were wounded in a fight between these groups of dealers.

The inhabitants of Christiania felt that the constant presence of armed police disrupted their lives, and cannabis smokers in Christiania felt that they were being monitored by the police.[26] The relationship between the police and cannabis smokers and inhabitants of Christiania was therefore often tense, particularly when the revision of the Law on Euphoria-Inducing Substances came into force in June 2004, and possession of cannabis for personal use became a crime. *Jyllands-Posten* in particular reported on how, in June and July 2004, the police implemented a policy of zero tolerance towards cannabis smokers in Christiania, by searching them and imposing fines for smoking cannabis as well as for possession of small amounts of the drug (several offences have to be recorded before an individual is taken to court for possession of cannabis). As discussed earlier, there is a historical connection between cannabis smoking and life in Christiania, and Pusher Street and cannabis dealing were often discussed there in the context of government plans to close down the Free City. Many of the inhabitants did not therefore publicly oppose the closure of Pusher Street or the zero tolerance policy towards cannabis smokers, not only because they did not support the existence of Pusher Street, but also in an attempt to save Christiania as an alternative society.[27]

One year later: the cannabis market in Copenhagen

In Christiania, one year after the closing down of Pusher Street and despite the subsequent police activity, cannabis dealing and use – according to all three newspapers, press releases from the police and the author's observations – continue. However, dealing does not take place in public, and those who smoke cannabis hide it when the police are in the neighbourhood. Yet Pusher Street was only one of a number of places where cannabis could be bought in Copenhagen, and after it was closed, the cannabis market dispersed to other parts of the city, and some new sales methods were reported, such as dealing from cars or via the Internet. Previous dealing methods, especially hash clubs and street-level dealing, were given renewed attention by the three newspapers.

In September 2004, the head of the drug squad in Copenhagen reported that, of an estimated 30 hash clubs in the city, about 17 clubs had opened since the closing down of Pusher Street.[28] He added that the zero tolerance policy not only applied to Pusher Street, but would also be implemented for hash clubs.[29–30.] In February 2005, the newspapers reported that the police had begun organised actions against hash clubs, and in early March the head of the drug squad stated that there were less than ten such clubs left in Copenhagen.[31] Less than two weeks later, on the first anniversary of the closing down of Pusher Street, *Politiken* demolished the police perception of the hash club situation. On the front page of the paper there was a map of Copenhagen, with the addresses of more than 30 hash clubs, and two full pages were used to describe the situation, including the fact that over 20 of these clubs were unknown to the police.[32] *Politiken*'s aim was to show that the cannabis market remains well established, even though Pusher Street had been closed. Its editorial published on the same day described Denmark's drug policy as a 'fiasco', and maintained that cannabis dealing was now dispersed all over Copenhagen, rather than being concentrated on Pusher Street.

Politiken became a player in the drug policy debate by running an article that overtly criticised the work of the police and the basis for the present government's drug policy for tackling the cannabis market in Copenhagen. The article attracted so much attention that politicians from different parties asked the Minister of Justice for a review of the situation. The other two newspapers considered in this chapter found it necessary to state their opinion on the situation in their editorials. *Jyllands-Posten* emphasised that the present drug policy was necessary and must be continued, that the development of hash clubs after the closing down of Pusher Street was predictable, and that the police must now take actions against these clubs.[33,34] *Berlingske Tidende* also supported the drug policy and asked the police to destroy any cannabis market with all the means they had at their disposal.[35] In the aftermath of *Politiken*'s article, in an interview with the paper, the head of the drug squad in Copenhagen explained that raids and other actions had been made regularly by the police since the implementation of the Hash Club Law in 2001, and over 100 clubs had been closed.[36]

New and dispersed street-level cannabis dealing in Copenhagen first received newspaper attention in *Jyllands-Posten* in February 2005,[31,37] followed by *Politiken* in March of that year.[38,39] Street-level dealing was reported as a new phenomenon in areas across the city, although the papers' attention was focused on Enghave Plads, because in February 2005 a group of 150 citizens established the 'Night Owls', who organised patrols around their neighbourhood in areas where cannabis dealing had emerged since the closure of Pusher Street. The Night Owls' aim was to protect their teenage children from contact with cannabis dealers, whose dealing methods were described as pushy and aggressive. The group was especially worried about their children getting into debt with the dealers and therefore becoming dependent upon them. One of the founders of the Night Owls was interviewed in *Jyllands-Posten*[37] and said that he had lived in the area for 30 years, but had never before experienced such open cannabis dealing. He directly related this development to the closure of Pusher Street.

One of the themes relating to street-level cannabis dealing that was most often raised by all three newspapers was that it was conducted close to schools and youth clubs, so that schoolchildren and young teenagers were exposed to the drug and could easily obtain it. *Politiken* emphasised that the increased availability of cannabis to young teenagers was one of the harmful consequences that the new drug policy and the closure of Pusher Street had for ordinary citizens.[31] *Jyllands-Posten*, on the other hand, used the situation to call for more community policing.[40]

There are two main reasons why two forms of cannabis dealing – hash clubs and street-level dealing – were given special attention in the newspapers. First, hash clubs were portrayed by all three newspapers as the means by which a large proportion of cannabis is sold in Copenhagen. Thus when *Politiken* wanted to criticise Danish drug policy, it published a map of the locations of these hash clubs in the city, thereby drawing further attention to what was already perceived to be important. Secondly, street-level dealing and hash clubs are overt and visible, and therefore young children and teenagers are exposed to them and their parents cannot control this exposure. Concern about the possibility of children and young people becoming addicts is frequently used to argue for more repressive drug policies,[4] and it was shown earlier that the government's action plan on drug use[1] and the tightening and revision of relevant laws were based on this concern.

Conclusion

Drug policies, whether they are liberal or repressive, are interpretations of how drugs in general and drug problems in particular are understood. They are political declarations of intent and how this should be put into practice in law, as well as in more specific initiatives related to drug problems, such as treatment facilities and prevention strategies. Drug policies are also expressions of morality – what we will tolerate as a society, what we can accept, and what we will offer drug users, such as punishment or treatment. One of the primary intentions of the recent changes in Danish drug policy was to remove the distinction between 'soft' and 'hard' drugs, in order to 'tidy up' the cannabis market and thereby decrease the accessibility of cannabis. This aim was put into practice by closing Pusher Street in Christiania. The cannabis dealing that had been tolerated there for more than 30 years is now deemed intolerable. The Free City of Christiania is also no longer tolerated, and negotiations between Christiania and the government on 'legalisation' of the area are currently taking place.

One year after the closure of Pusher Street, there are disagreements about the cannabis market in Copenhagen. Community police, social workers and outreach workers claim that there is just as much cannabis circulating in Copenhagen as there was before the closure of Pusher Street, but that it has now dispersed to other and new locations.[41–43] They are the 'street-level bureaucrats'[26] whose job includes, among other things, remaining in contact with young people and keeping an eye on new trends in the drug market. Statistics from the Danish Board of Health also show that cannabis use did not decrease between 2004 and 2005[19,20] and, in an internal memo, Copenhagen Municipality concluded that up to 60% of the 16- to 19-year-olds in the city have tried the drug.[43] When interviewed in the three newspapers reviewed here, both cannabis users and dealers also claimed that cannabis remained easily accessible.[27,44] On the other hand, representatives of the Copenhagen drug squad – the police department that planned and implemented the closure of Pusher Street – have continued to claim that there is less distribution of cannabis in Copenhagen now than previously, although their main evidence for this is a decrease in the sale of cannabis to tourists.[42]

Of the different kinds of claim makers represented in the three newspapers, the police were most often used. Other claim makers (e.g. professionals, cannabis users and cannabis dealers) have experience and knowledge of the cannabis market in Copenhagen, but their voices were used relatively less often. With their choice of claim makers, the three newspapers also provide a particular view of the cannabis situation in Copenhagen. Although *Politiken* used the widest variety of claim makers and took an active political stand by criticising the work of the police one year after the closure of Pusher Street, it – like *Jyllands-Posten* and *Berlingske Tidende* – both initially supported the closure of Pusher Street and brought hash clubs and street-level dealing to public attention using the same issue as the other two newspapers, namely concern about the possibility of young people being exposed to drugs. In that sense, the three newspapers report on the case from the same standpoint – that drugs, including cannabis, are society's 'enemy',[13] and that young people in particular can become victims of them. They also put forward the same perception of drug policy, in particular that there is no difference between 'hard' and 'soft' drugs, or between users and dealers. Since the three newspapers represent different political perspectives, one could conclude that the dominant discourse on drugs in Denmark in general has moved towards a less liberal understanding of drug problems. The morality that forms the basis of repressive drug policies therefore seems to be more generally accepted in Danish society at large, and is not just the perspective of the present government.

Other studies have shown that repressive drug policies have little effect on drug markets, despite increased police efforts to eliminate those markets.[7,8] In relation to the cannabis market in Copenhagen, the conclusion must be that the intended aim of the changes to a more repressive drug policy has failed. The police actions have had little effect on the size of the cannabis market, and have only dispersed it to new locations in the city.

References

1 Ministry of Home Affairs and Ministry of Health. *The Fight Against Drugs: action plan against drug misuse.* Copenhagen: Ministry of Home Affairs and Ministry of Health; 2003.

2 Storgaard LL. Trends in cannabis use and changes in cannabis policy in Denmark. In: Kraus L, Korf DJ, editors. *Research on Drugs and Drug Policy from a European Perspective.* Munich: Pabst Science Publishers; 2005.

3 Balvig F, Rasmussen N. *Visse sider af forholdet mellem befolkningen, Christiania og politiet [Perspectives on the Relationship Between the Public, Christiania and the Police].* Copenhagen: Kriminalistisk Instituts Stecilserie no. 25; 1984.

4 Laursen L. Scandinavia's tug of war on drugs. In: Hakkarainen P, Laursen L, Tigerstedt C, editors. *Discussing Drugs and Control Policy. Comparative studies on four Nordic countries.* Helsinki: NAD Publications No. 31; 1996.

5 Lauritsen PW. *Christiania: kort fortalt guide og historie [Christiania: a brief guide and history].* Copenhagen: Aschehoug; 2002.

6 Asmussen V. *Cannabis Dealers and Private Security Guards: an example of the recent changes in Danish drug policy.* EMCDDA monograph. Lisbon: European Monitoring Centre for Drugs and Drug Addition.

7 Kilmer B. Do cannabis possession laws influence cannabis use? In: *Cannabis 2002 Report. Technical Report of the International Scientific Conference.* Brussels, Belgium, 25 February 2001.

8 Korf D. Dutch coffee shops and trends in cannabis use. *Addict Behav.* 2002; **27**: 851–66.

9 Balvig F. *Kriminalitet og Social Kontrol [Crime and Social Control].* Copenhagen: Columbus; 1999.

10 Asmussen V, Moesby-Johansen C. The legal response to illegal 'hash clubs' in Denmark. In: Decorte T, Korf D, editors. *European Studies on Drugs and Drug Policy.* Brussels: VUB Press; 2004.

11 www.infomedia.dk

12 Spector M, Kitsuse JI. *Constructing Social Problems.* New York: Aldine De Gruyter; 1987.

13 Christie N, Bruun K. *Den Gode Fiende. Narkotikapolitikk i Norden [The Good Enemy. Drug policy in the Nordic countries].* Oslo: Universitetsforlaget; 1985.

14 Law Prohibiting Visitors to Designated Places Act of 2001, No. 471; www.retsinfo.dk

15 Law on Euphoria-Inducing Substances Act of 2004, No. 445; www.retsinfo.dk

16 Prison Law Act of 2004, No. 445; www.retsinfo.dk

17 www.retsinfo.dk

18 EMCDDA. *Annual Report. The state of the drugs problem in the European Union and Norway.* Lisbon: EMCDDA; 2004.

19 Focal Point. *Narkotikasituation i Danmark [The Drug Situation in Denmark].* Copenhagen: Sundhedsstyrelsen; 2004.

20 Focal Point. *Narkotikasituation i Danmark [The Drug Situation in Denmark].* Copenhagen: Sundhedsstyrelsen; 2005.

21 Suskiewicz F, Olesen L, Barsøe M et al., editors. *Christiania på arbejde. Statusrapport: Fra vision til virkelighed. [Christiania at Work. Progress report: from vision to reality].* Copenhagen: Christiania; 2003.

22 Christianias Baggrundsgruppe [Christiania's Background Group]. *Christiania: en hvidbog i farver [Christiania: a white paper in colour].* Copenhagen: Christiania; 2005.

23 Jæger B, Olesen L, Rieper O. *De offentlige myndigheder og Christiania [The Public Authorities and Christiania].* Copenhagen: AKF Forlaget; 1993.

24 Building and Housing Administration of Copenhagen. *En mulig vej for Christiania: som fond og almen boligorganisation [A Possible Way for Christiania: as a foundation and common housing organisation].* Copenhagen: KAB; 2004.

25 Christianiaudvalget [The Christiania Committee]. *Christianiaområdets fremtid: helhedsplan og handlingsplan [Christiania's Future: an action plan].* Copenhagen: Christianiaudvalget; 2004.

26 Lipsky M. *Street-Level Bureaucracy. Dilemmas of the individual in public services.* New York: Russell Sage Foundation; 1980.

27 *Jyllands-Posten*, 28 January 2005.

28 *Berlingske Tidende*, 6 September 2004.

29 *Jyllands-Posten*, 19 March 2004.

30 *Politiken*, 18 February 2005.

31 *Jyllands-Posten*, 4 March 2005.

32 *Politiken*, 16 March 2005.

33 *Jyllands-Posten*, 17 March 2005.

34 *Jyllands-Posten*, 26 March 2005.

35 *Berlingske Tidende*, 17 March 2005.

36 *Politiken*, 27 March 2005.

37 *Jyllands-Posten*, 22 February 2005.

38 *Politiken*, 20 March 2005.

39 *Politiken*, 26 March 2005.

40 *Jyllands-Posten*, 1 March 2005.

41 *Jyllands-Posten*, 18 June 2005.
42 *Berlingske Tidende*, 5 June 2005.
43 Municipality of Copenhagen. Internal memo. 25 May 2005.
44 *Politiken*, 18 March 2005.

Chapter 3

Characteristics of the cannabis market in Belgium

Tom Decorte

Over the past few years, the evolution of the cannabis market in Belgium has been frequently commented upon in a wide range of publications.[1-4] The number of cannabis plantations uncovered by the Belgian judiciary has been rising steadily, and the relocation of cannabis production to the Low Countries (i.e. Belgium and the Netherlands) has often been associated with a growing professionalisation of its cultivation and the involvement of organised crime, and with a more noxious and hazardous product compared with cannabis imported from elsewhere (due to a higher concentration of the most psychoactive chemical in cannabis, delta-9-tetrahydrocannabinol or THC, and thus a stronger potency, and to the presence of remnants of pesticides and other toxic chemicals).

After briefly considering the patterns of cannabis use in Belgium and the current policy in relation to the drug, this chapter describes some characteristics of cannabis supply and attempts to unravel its complex relationship with current government policy. In order to understand some of the changes that the Belgian cannabis market has undergone in recent years, important features and developments in the Dutch cannabis market must also be considered. Belgium and the Netherlands not only share a border which is easily crossed in the context of the European Union, but they are also historically connected. In the twelfth century, towns grew up in the region of *de Nederlanden* – low-lying land around the deltas of the Rhine, Scheldt and Meuse (Maas) rivers. Today, the Low Countries share many similarities. For example, the population of northern Belgium, the Flemish, speak the same language as the Dutch. Moreover, as there are multiple forms of legal cooperation at a political, economic and cultural level, it must be assumed that there are also multiple forms of illegal cross-border cooperation and influences.

Cannabis use in Belgium

Centuries ago, large parts of Flanders and the Netherlands were covered with hemp fields.[5] The hemp seed was used as a food grain and the fibres were used to make rope, sail and canvas, clothes, shoes and paper.[6] In the course of the twentieth century, the industrial hemp plant disappeared from the fields, under the influence of an ideological and political climate that was increasingly hostile to the cultivation of hemp plants, in the context of moral panic over the negative consequences of recreational cannabis use in the USA and elsewhere, even though most varieties of industrial hemp had a low THC content. In the mid-twentieth century, in the aftermath of American activity against the 'killer weed', hemp cultivation was prohibited practically everywhere in the world. Around the same time, cannabis increased in popularity as an intoxicating and pleasurable substance. In the 1940s and 1950s, American soldiers and jazz musicians acquainted their European fellow soldiers and musicians with the reefer. Poets, writers and visual artists started to smoke 'hash' (cannabis resin) and 'weed' (the dried flowers of the cannabis plant), while immigrants, including those from former colonies, introduced the cultural use of cannabis to the countries where they settled.[6]

The image and function of cannabis have changed during the last few decades.[4] In the 1960s, the use of cannabis increased in artistic circles and in the counter-culture movement, but was mainly confined to subcultures, whereas now cannabis is used by members of all social strata, and its use has become part of the general (but particularly youth) culture. The Belgian government has always maintained that its drug policy has never implied that drug use in society could become 'normal', but despite this policy and its concomitant predominantly repressive discourse, the use of cannabis has become more widespread in Belgium, as well as more open to public discussion. A significant proportion of the population, particularly young people, have adopted a tolerant attitude towards cannabis use that is not unlike that towards the use of alcohol and legal medicines. In the light of what has been taking place in other countries, this development is unsurprising. Cannabis is the most widely used, produced and traded illegal substance worldwide, and its 'normalisation' has occurred in most European countries.[7] It therefore appears that patterns of cannabis use have changed independently and cannot easily be influenced by any national policy.[8,9]

With regard to the actual number of cannabis users in Belgium, to date there have been no accurate national prevalence surveys among the adult population. It was not until 2001 that the Belgian National Health Survey included some questions on drug use and showed that 10.8% of the national adult population aged 15–64 years had used cannabis at some point in their life, and 2.8% had used it during the last month.[10] The first European School Survey Project on Alcohol and Other Drugs (ESPAD), undertaken in Belgium in 2003, showed that 32.2% of the school population aged 15–16 years had used cannabis at least once in their life, and 16.7% had used it during the last month.[11] Although these indicators are indirect and incomplete, media sources, political and scientific opinion makers and drug experts all agree that the use of cannabis has become more widespread.

Cannabis policy in Belgium

The drug policy document that the Belgian federal government (a socialist–liberal coalition) approved in 2001 expressed the political will to stop prosecuting people for using cannabis on condition that this use was 'non-problematic and not causing nuisance' and 'personal' only.[12] The same applied to the cultivation of cannabis – nothing more than an anonymous police record would be effected under these conditions. This record would be made solely for the purpose of mapping the drug phenomenon, and, it was argued, as it would not contain any information on the identity of the individual caught in possession of or growing cannabis, they could not be prosecuted or cautioned. The approval of this federal policy document, which can be regarded as an official declaration of intent, was followed by two years of pervasive uncertainty and legal insecurity concerning what was effectively permitted, as the Narcotic Drug Act of 1921 was not altered by Parliament until 4 April and 3 May 2003. Following the Ministerial Circular of 16 March 2003 on 'The prosecution policy with regard to the possession of and the retail trade in illegal narcotic substances', which replaced the previous guidelines of 1998, the possession of 3 grams of cannabis and the cultivation of cannabis for 'personal use' (that is, one female cannabis plant) is no longer grounds for prosecution. In the case of larger amounts, the public prosecutor may, in principle, intervene and prosecute the grower. Thus it remains unclear whether prosecutions will be brought against, for example, an individual who has grown three or four cannabis plants, a grower who imports seeds or cuttings from another country, or the owner of a plant that yields more than 3 grams of cannabis.

The supply of cannabis

Until the late 1960s, cannabis (particularly hash) was imported into Belgium from Afghanistan, Pakistan, India and Nepal, and later also from Lebanon and Morocco. There was little organised wholesale trade, the hash being smuggled and distributed mainly by holidaymakers and travellers (many of whom used the drug themselves) through a variety of channels and in relatively small quantities. Occasionally, cargoes of weed were imported from Indonesia, Thailand, Colombia and Jamaica.

In the late 1960s and especially in the 1970s, important changes in the cannabis market in the Netherlands took place, which affected the cannabis market in Belgium. The Dutch police and judiciary paid particular attention to the trafficking in so-called 'hard drugs', which initially meant heroin, but later also cocaine. Some shipments of cannabis were seized, but its detection was given only low priority.[13] However, there were some illegal entrepreneurs who saw an opportunity to expand their activities, which they focused on the more profitable export of locally grown cannabis to other countries, including Belgium. More illegal entrepreneurs were attracted by the money to be made, and when those involved in more organised crime gangs arrived on the scene, the illegal hash trade became bigger and more commercial, with more links to other criminal activities (such as money laundering and prostitution), and it also became more violent. By the late 1980s, a number of 'hash barons' had appointed themselves as main players. Probably the best known among them was Klaas Bruinsma, who was gunned down in 1991.[14,15] This gangland killing marked the beginning of a surge of murders that coloured the Dutch underworld, and which without exception involved individuals who had made a fortune in the hash trade. The judicial investigations into these traffickers discovered that they had branched out into the criminal underworld in Belgium and also in many other countries.

Foreign methods of investigation in the Low Countries

Meanwhile, investigation and detection techniques in Belgium, as in other countries, had become Americanised, inspired by the US 'War on Drugs.' Since the second half of the 1960s, American legal attachés had exerted a deliberate influence on the fight against crime in various ways and in diverse areas.[16,17] The American Drug Enforcement Administration (DEA), who enforce the US federal controlled substances laws, increasingly expanded its activities abroad from the late 1970s onwards. Through educational courses and conferences, Belgian law enforcement officers were familiarised with special criminal investigation methods, including pseudo-purchases, controlled shipments, infiltration and civilian informants.[18] This American influence on investigation and detection methods resulted in high-profile convictions of members of the Belgian National Drugs Bureau[19] for drugs trafficking and falsifying and destroying documents with fraudulent intent. It also discredited the head of the

Brussels Judiciary Police[18] for improper methods of investigation inspired by American police officers, and also led to a parliamentary inquiry and the resignation of ministers in the Netherlands over controlled shipments of cannabis without permission from a higher authority.

Domestic cannabis: from *nederweed* (Dutch cannabis) to 'euroweed'

Whereas in the 1960s and 1970s the Belgian cannabis market was supplied mainly by foreign sources, a major shift towards domestic (i.e. locally grown) cannabis began in the early 1980s. This domestic cannabis was grown both by individual users (on a small scale, usually at home) and by commercial entrepreneurs (on a large scale, and professionally managed). As the 'War on Drugs' intensified under President Reagan, some Americans (including 'Sam the Skunkman') settled in the Netherlands, which became an incubation environment for the indoor cultivation of cannabis plants.[20] New cultivation, crossbreeding and cloning techniques gave rise to many new forms of a seedless variety (sensimilla) that were of a higher quality than the original native weed.

The increase in domestic cultivation was aided by the existence of 'coffee shops', where the selling of cannabis for personal consumption by the public has been tolerated by the local authorities under the drug policy of the Netherlands since 1976. However, these coffee shops illustrate the ongoing contradiction in the Dutch policy, as they are allowed to sell cannabis, but not to buy it. Coffee shops needed a constant and undisrupted supply, and were willing to buy crops from local growers. Domestic cultivation was further stimulated by the increasing demand for Dutch cannabis because of its reputedly superior quality, the flexibility displayed by local growers in response to demand, and the spread of 'grow shops' (that sell the paraphernalia for growing cannabis) throughout the country.[21] Although in the early 1990s the coffee shops were still selling weed from Colombia, Thailand, Jamaica and Nigeria, the Dutch-grown 'skunk' proved to be much more popular. The older generation of cannabis traders were joined by newcomers – those in their twenties who were primarily focused on growing, rather than selling imported weed.[22] The fact that these developments in the Netherlands were soon followed by similar trends in Belgium is unsurprising, given the links between the two countries described earlier, the almost non-existent border controls in a European free market, and the location of some of the Dutch coffee shops only a few kilometres away from the Belgian border. The Dutch expertise in domestic cultivation techniques was thus readily exported, while at the same time many

Belgian cannabis users travelled regularly to the Netherlands to obtain their supplies. The shift from foreign to domestic cannabis on the Belgian market is reflected in the police statistics, although these are rather scarce and often inconsistent. The police journal *Pol* reports that Belgian cannabis production increased by 400% between 1996 and 2000, while the number of plantations seized by the police rose from 63 in 1996 to 730 in 1999.

The present development of the Belgian cannabis market can be called a process of 'import substitution', in which the share of imported cannabis is decreasing steadily and that of locally cultivated cannabis is increasing steeply. It concurs perfectly with the international trend. In North America (e.g. California) and in British Columbia, Canada, large-scale cultivation (both indoor and outdoor) has become established. While the Netherlands has long played a pioneering role in cannabis cultivation in Western Europe, local cultivation has also increased in Switzerland, Spain, Belgium, the UK, Albania and other Eastern European countries.[23,24] The large numbers of cannabis fairs and grow shops in various countries testify to this trend.

Domestic cultivation: professionalism and criminal organisations

Simultaneously with the trend in import substitution, as described above, the logistics of the cannabis trade have changed dramatically in the last two decades. The wholesale trade in imported hash often used to involve large bulk shipments, but with expanding local cultivation, the scale of the supply has become significantly smaller. However, the precise ratio of small-scale production to professional large-scale production in this illicit sector has not yet been established.

A study by criminologist Bovenkerk[25] caused a great deal of controversy in the Netherlands, as its conclusions highlighted the professionalism and organisational resources behind the plantations that had been discovered by the police. According to Bovenkerk, hemp cultivation had reached a stage far beyond personal gardening and had become a matter of organised crime, particularly in areas of social deprivation where inhabitants were being put under pressure to make their homes available for cultivation (*leasekweek*). Bovenkerk further concluded that although theoretically the far-reaching regularisation of hemp cultivation by the government would be the most appropriate course of action, in practice this was unfeasible in an international context, and a more consistently repressive position would eventually be inevitable. There may be no causal relationship, but shortly after this study was published, the Dutch judiciary started to act more forcefully against cannabis cultivation.

Bovenkerk's most important recommendation, which was to investigate and prosecute the organisations behind the cannabis production and trafficking, rather than to punish smaller growers, has been followed little if at all so far. On the contrary, the police and the judiciary, together with electricity companies and housing associations, now take a firm line on home growing. Now that people can be evicted from their homes if they are caught growing weed, many small growers have stopped producing cannabis. However, this may actually stimulate larger-scale and more criminal cultivation. At the end of 2005, many coffee shop managers were complaining about the rising prices of Dutch weed, which might have been a consequence of a drop in supply. They also found it more difficult to get hold of organically grown weed from small home growers.[26]

The discourse about the criminal nature of domestic cannabis cultivation has regularly been accompanied by public concern about increasing THC levels in the drug, the use of pesticides and the possible relationship between the use of this strong and/or polluted cannabis and the development of mental disorders. Pesticides used in ornamental plant cultivation were found in a number of marijuana samples in 2001 in the Netherlands.[27] Furthermore, the average THC level in *nederweed* doubled from 9% in 2000 to 18% in 2003.[28] This was a reason from some to argue in favour of classifying this potent cannabis as a 'hard drug.' In Belgium, seized cannabis samples were analysed by the Scientific Institute of Public Health in collaboration with the Office of the Public Prosecutor in Antwerp in 2004, when the average THC level was found to be 13.2% in marijuana and 14% in hash.

The discourse on the involvement of the criminal underworld in the production of *nederweed* has reached Belgium in recent years. Fed by statements from police experts and politicians, the media have been painting a picture of exponentially expanding cannabis cultivation that is increasingly professional because it is in the hands of organised criminal groups. Criminal control over cannabis cultivation is often portrayed in the Belgian media in terms of the increasing use of pesticides, artificially high THC levels, the taking over of private homes and even whole housing estates in order to grow cannabis, the installation of booby traps to protect plantations against trespassers, and the use of cannabis as currency among criminals.

The expansion of cannabis cultivation in Belgium appears to be partly a consequence of the stricter treatment to which cannabis cultivation has been subjected in the Netherlands. According to media reports, the increased levels of cannabis cultivation in Belgium have been further boosted by the Dutch grow shops, which offer new growers all the necessary equipment very cheaply or sometimes in exchange for a part of the yield of the first harvests. This may lead to an absurd situation in which Belgian 'drug tourists' travel to Dutch coffee shops in order to stock up with *Belgoweed* seeds that are grown in Belgium and then exported to the Netherlands.

Police statistics show that in Belgium the number of plantations that have been dismantled by the authorities has increased sharply in recent years, although it must be noted that as few as two or three plants constitute a 'plantation' according to the law. Although illicit cultivation is found in nearly every police district in Belgium, it appears to be most heavily concentrated in the eastern and north-eastern areas at the Dutch border. Cannabis is being cultivated not only more frequently, but also on a larger scale. According to the police, the large-scale plantations in Belgium (that is, those comprising more than 500 plants, often spread over several rooms, and with automatic or computer-controlled technology) involve a strikingly large number of Dutch citizens – as organisers, growers or suppliers of materials. However, the police data on cannabis cultivation that are available in Belgium not only show little consistency, but may also have been influenced at least indirectly by the particular investigation activities and priorities of the local police and judiciary, the growing media focus on cannabis cultivation, changes in legislation and criminal law policy, and citizens' willingness to report cannabis cultivation. Thus although large-scale cultivation of cannabis in the Belgian border area with the Netherlands has increased under the influence of Dutch professional growers, it cannot be explained only by influences emanating from the Netherlands. Moreover, small-scale and/or non-commercial cannabis cultivation in Belgium has not been documented.

In Belgium, as in numerous other countries, there is a significant demand for cannabis, and the product appears to have established itself as a 'normal' consumer product among the younger generation. According to spokespeople of the Dutch grow shops, the Drugs Policy Document of the Belgian federal government and the changes in legislation that it entailed initially resulted in a rush of Belgian citizens who wished to start growing their own supplies. Interviews that the Institute for Social Drug Research is currently conducting with cannabis growers show that many of them are enthusiastic amateur growers (rather than large-scale growers), who consider their own grown cannabis to be a cheaper and better alternative to that purchased elsewhere.[24] A study of 369 experienced cannabis users in Belgium showed that 59% of them had acquired cannabis through friends, and less than one in four respondents had purchased cannabis in one or more coffee shops in the Netherlands.[3] The same study showed that 7% of the respondents were themselves growing cannabis at the time of the interview, and that nearly a third (30%) had tried to grow one or more cannabis plants at home at least once.[4,29]

Conclusion

In the last 40 years, the cannabis market in Belgium (and in other European countries) has undergone a major development, described in this chapter as a process of import substitution. Whereas until the late 1980s the market had been supplied by bulk import of foreign cannabis (hash), domestic cultivation gradually increased in importance with the advent of new growing techniques and crossbred varieties. This shift towards (inter-)regional production, trade and domestic cultivation has also been found in North America and Western and Eastern Europe, and appears to be irreversible. It is not inconceivable that more recent experiments with *skuff* or *nederhash* (which is manufactured from weed through a pollinator) herald the beginning of the domestic production of cannabis resin (hash), as some users prefer this to weed.

During the same period, the image and function of cannabis have also changed completely. Among a significant proportion of the population (particularly young people) it has become a subject of open debate and its use has become acceptable, regardless of drug policy. Whereas in the Netherlands, at the instigation of dozens of mayors, there are increasing calls for better regulation of the supply of cannabis to the coffee shops, in Belgium there are increasing demands (by police departments among others) for the control of domestic cannabis cultivation to become a national priority. Little thought has been given to the effects that a more repressive enforcement may have on market organisation, the growing techniques and the quality of the cannabis products. Moreover, preliminary questions that have not been answered include the proportion of the market that is supplied by small producers and by larger producers involved in organised crime, the proportion of the Belgian market that is still being supplied with products imported by wholesalers, and the proportion of domestic production that is exported to neighbouring countries and further abroad.

Finally, some thought should be given to the question of whether decriminalisation of the possession of small quantities of cannabis and the tolerance of growing small quantities of the drug would, in a European context, not be more effective than the Dutch coffee shop model (which, in the author's view, is an inconsistent combination of tolerating possession and use of small quantities, but prohibiting the production and supply of cannabis), or constitute a compromise between the extremes of outright commercialisation and unqualified decriminalisation of possession and use. If users are thus offered the opportunity to supply themselves with their product, the detection and penalisation of large-scale and heavily commercialised cultivation (which is often more hazardous to the consumer's health) remains perfectly possible.

References

1 De Ruyver B, Casselman J, Meuwissen K *et al. Het Belgisch Drugbeleid Anno 2000: een stand van zaken drie jaar na de aanbevelingen van de parlementaire werkgroep drugs [Belgian Drug Policy for the Year 2000: a state of the art three years after the recommendations of the parliamentary commission on drugs].* Ghent: University of Ghent, Onderzoeksgroep Drugbeleid, Strafrechtelijk Beleid en Internationale Criminaliteit; 2000.

2 Vander Laene F. *Drugbeleid op School: de leerlingen aan het woord [Drug Policy at School: the perspective of the pupils].* Ghent: Institute for International Research on Criminal Policy; 2003.

3 Vereniging voor alcohol en andere drugproblemen. *Visie op Cannabis Vanuit de Gespecialiseerde Drugsector [Perspectives on Cannabis from the Drug Expert Sector].* Brussels: VAD; 2000.

4 Decorte T, Muys M, Slock S. *Cannabis in Vlaanderen: patronen van cannabisgebruik bij ervaren gebruikers [Cannabis in Flanders: patterns of use among experienced users].* Leuven: Uitgeverij Acco; 2003.

5 Lindemans P. *De Geschiedenis van de Landbouw in België [History of Agriculture in Belgium].* Antwerp: Genootschap voor Geschiedenis en Volkskunde; 1994.

6 Van Scharen H. *De Cannabis Connectie [The Cannabis Connection].* Antwerp: Uitgeverij Hadewijch; 1997.

7 European Monitoring Centre for Drugs and Drug Addiction (EMCDDA). *Annual Report 2004: the state of the drugs problem in the European Union and Norway.* Lisbon: EMCDDA; 2004.

8 Korf D. Dutch coffee shops and trends in cannabis use. *Addict Behav.* 2002; **27**: 851–66.

9 Cohen P, Kaal H. *The Irrelevance of Drug Policy. Patterns and careers of experienced cannabis use in the populations of Amsterdam, San Francisco and Bremen.* Amsterdam: Centre for Drug Research; 2001.

10 Gisle L, Buziarsist J, Van der Heyden J et al. *Gezondheidsenquête door Middel van Interview (HIS), België 2001 [National Health Survey Through Interviews, Belgium 2001].* Brussels: Wetenschappelijk Instituut Volksgezondheid; 2002.

11 Lambrecht P, Andries C, Engels T *et al. ESPAD 03: Outline for Belgian Report 2. Results for Belgium 2003.* Brussels: Vrije Universiteit Brussel; 2004.

12 *Beleidsnota van de Federale Regering in Verband met de drugproblematiek [Policy Declaration on the Drug Problem by the Federal Government], Brussels, 19 January 2001*; www.minsoc.fgov.be/cabinet/2001_01_19_federale_beleidsnota_drugs.htm# fede-ralenota

13 van Es K. *De Coffeeshop. De opmerkelijke geschiedenis van een Hollands fenomeen [The Coffee Shop. The remarkable history of a Dutch phenomenon].* Amsterdam: Mets; 1997.

14 Klerks P. *Groot in de Hasj. Theorie en praktijk van de georganiseerde criminaliteit [Big in Hash. Theory and practice in organised crime].* Antwerp: Kluwer; 2000.

15 Middelburg B. *De Godmother. De criminele carrière van Thea Moear, medeoprichter van de Bruinsma groep [The Godmother. The criminal career of Thea Moear, co-founder of the Bruinsma group].* Amsterdam: Veen; 2000.

16 Nadelmann E. *Cops Across Borders. The internationalization of US criminal law enforcement.* University Park, PA: Pennsylvania State Press; 1993.

17 Hoogenboom B. The eagle has landed (2). *Tijdschr Politie.* 1996; **10**: 11–15.

18 Decorte T, Van Laethem W. *Grijze Politie. Verklaringen voor problematische publiek–private interacties in de zaak-Reyniers [Grey Policing. Explanations for*

problematic public–private interactions in the Reyniers case]. Brussels: Uitgeverij Politeia; 1997.

19 Raes F. *Rijkswachter als Don Quichot. Een B.O.B.'er op speurtocht bij het Nationaal Bureau voor Drugs [A Special Agent as Don Quixote. A special agent investigating the National Bureau on Drugs]*. Berchem: Uitgeverij EPO; 1983.

20 Jansen M. Prijsvorming in de Nederlandse marihuana sector 1990–1995: een beleidsperspectief [Price setting in the Dutch marijuana sector 1990–1995: a policy perspective]. *Economisch Statistische Berichten*, 20 March 1996.

21 Jansen M. Het succes van de Nederlandse marijuanateelt [The success of Dutch marijuana cultivation]. *Econ Stat Berichten*. 1996; **81**: 257–9.

22 Korf D, Verbraeck H. *Dealers en Dienders. Dynamiek tussen drugsbestrijding en de midden- en hogere niveaus van de cannabis-, cocaïne-, amfetamine en ecstasyhandel in Amsterdam [Dealers and Bureaucrats. Dynamics between drug enforcement and the middle and higher levels of the cannabis, cocaine, amphetamine and MDMA trade in Amsterdam]*. Amsterdam: 'Bonger' Institute of Criminology, University of Amsterdam; 1993.

23 Jansen M. De economie van de cannabissector in beleidsperspectief [The economy of the cannabis sector from a policy perspective]. *Econ Stat Berichten*. 2002; **4354**: 276–8.

24 Hough M, Warburton H, Few B *et al*. *A Growing Market: the domestic cultivation of cannabis*. York: Joseph Rowntree Foundation; 2003.

25 Bovenkerk F, Hogewind W. *Hennepteelt in Nederland: het probleem van de criminaliteit en haar bestrijding [Hemp Cultivation in The Netherlands: the problem of crime and its enforcement]*. Utrecht: Willem Pompe Instituut voor Strafwetenschappen/Apeldoorn: Politie en Wetenschap; 2002.

26 Stoke E, Uitham R. Geen liefde voor het plantje [No love for the plant]. *De Volkskrant (De Voorkant)*, 9 December 2005.

27 Traag A, Gercek H, Kloet D *et al*. *Onderzoek naar Residuen van Bestrijdingsmiddelen in Nederwiet [Study of Residues of Pesticides in Dutch Weed]*. Utrecht: Trimbos Institute; 2001.

28 Niesink M, Pijlman F, Righter S. *THC-concentraties in wiet, nederwiet en hasj in Nederlandse coffeeshops (2002–2003) [Concentrations of THC in weed, Dutch weed and hash in Dutch coffee shops (2002–2003]*. Utrecht: Trimbos Institute; 2003.

29 Decorte T, Tuteleers P. *Cannabisteelt in Vlaanderen [Cannabis cultivation in Flanders]*. Unpublished paper. See also www.law.ugent.be/crim/ISD

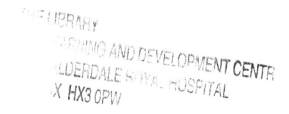

Chapter 4

Ephedra for fun, performance and losing weight

Cas Barendregt and Brigitte Boon

Substances that contain ephedra are known to aid weight loss and enhance athletic performance.[1] Until April 2004 in the Netherlands, products containing this substance were available in pharmacies but also in so-called 'smart shops' (establishments where legal psychoactive substances are sold, usually for leisure purposes), where they were marketed as drugs for recreational use.[2] On 6 April 2004, the Dutch government classified ephedra alkaloids as a medical drug in the Act on the Provision of Medical Drugs. This has led to a de facto ban on their sales.[3] It is unlikely that ephedra alkaloids will become officially registered as a regular medicinal drug, because their primary effects serve no medical purpose. Ephedra contains two active ingredients, ephedrine and pseudo-ephedrine, both of which stimulate the autonomic nervous system in the same way as the endogenous neurotransmitter adrenaline. In Europe, these substances are classified as precursors[4] – that is, substances which, following a chemical reaction when mixed with other substances, become an intrinsic part of a new product. As precursors, ephedrine and pseudo-ephedrine are used to produce the synthetic stimulant drug methamphetamine.

Ephedra is a generic term for a number of extracts from ephedra-containing herbs that are known under their Chinese name *Ma huang*. As a traditional medicine, ephedra was used as a bronchodilator to treat asthmatic complaints.[5] Ephedra is a substance that, when swallowed, acts as an amphetamine-like stimulant. As a crude product it commonly occurs in the form of fine grains, but for retail purposes it is usually mixed with other substances, such as caffeine, and sold in tablet form. Simultaneous use with caffeine or aspirin increases the effect of ephedra.[6]

The use of ephedra may have negative effects on health. There are indications that even small quantities of ephedra alkaloids may increase the risk of hypertension, stroke, myocardial infarction (heart attack) and psychosis.[7-11] Moreover, the combination of ephedra with caffeine or aspirin may increase some health risks, such as the development of psychiatric symptoms and cardiovascular disease.[1,12]

Much of our knowledge of ephedra is based on medically oriented studies from the USA. In the Netherlands (and in the rest of Europe), no social studies on ephedra use have been published. Therefore the purpose of the exploratory study reported here was twofold – to explore the behaviour and perceptions of a self-selected sample of Dutch ephedra users and, one year after the official ban on ephedra use in the Netherlands, to document its impact on these users.

Methods

Semi-structured interviews were conducted with six managers or employees of smart shops. In addition, one expert from the pharmacy sector was interviewed. The information that emerged from these interviews provided some insight into the general features of the ephedra market and the impact of the ban on ephedra use. This information was used to develop an online questionnaire.

In March and April 2005, a structured pre-coded Internet questionnaire was administered online. Respondents were recruited via announcements on various Internet sites. Calls for participation and direct hyperlinks to the questionnaire were posted on discussion forums of two sites concerned with losing body weight, three techno-party sites and three drug information sites, two of which are operated by drug prevention professionals. Two advertisements were placed on the most popular Dutch advertisement websites in the categories 'sport and fitness' and 'contact and messages', and a press release was posted on a body-building site. Flyers in the form of small business cards were placed on the counters of eight smart shops, and posters inviting people to participate were put up in three smart shops. The smart shops that participated in the study were located in Rotterdam, Leiden, Eindhoven, Roermond and Maastricht. It was decided not to include smart shops in Amsterdam in the study, since most of their clients are probably not representative of the Dutch population, but are more likely to be tourists from other countries.

The questionnaire asked for demographic data, frequency of ephedra use (lifetime, recent and current), quantity of use, and the frequency of use of other psychoactive substances, including substitutes for ephedra. Responses to questions on reasons for use, the effects of use, and control over use were measured on a 5-point Likert scale. In addition to the pre-coded questions, respondents were also invited to make additional comments in free-text boxes.

In addition to the Internet questionnaire, 11 ephedra users were interviewed using a semi-structured interview schedule. The results of these interviews served to validate the data that emerged from the Internet questionnaire. Nine interviewees were selected from the Internet sample and two were recruited via an Internet advertisement. The criteria for selection were based on reasons for using ephedra, reported health complaints and body mass index (BMI) (a measure of the degree to which a person is underweight or overweight). Several respondents within each category of reasons for using ephedra that were indicated in the literature were interviewed. These categories were losing weight, improving performance and going out/having fun. Unfortunately, only a few of the respondents who reported health problems were willing to provide their email addresses, and none of them agreed to participate in a face-to-face interview.

Results

Of the 306 ephedra users who completed the questionnaire, 304 appeared to be valid and suitable for analysis. This section presents the results of the study in terms of the characteristics of the respondents, their use of ephedra and other drugs, their reasons for using ephedra, the reported effects of use of this drug and the health problems associated with it (including dependency), and changes in consumption patterns since the ban on sales, including the use of substitutes for ephedra.

Characteristics of the respondents

The 304 ephedra users whose data were included in the study were relatively young and well educated. Around 75% of the respondents to the Internet questionnaire were aged 30 years or younger (mean 26 years), and almost 50% of them were female. There was no significant difference in BMI between male and female respondents.* Less than 1% of the respondents were of non-Dutch origin, around 40% had received an average or high level of education, and 20% had received a low level of education. A third of the sample were studying or participating in some kind of professional training, and 63% were employed or worked on a freelance basis. Of the total sample, 3% were receiving social benefit or an invalidity pension. Almost 50% of the respondents lived with a partner, and about 50% had one or more children.

Ephedra use

For 53% of the sample, initiation into ephedra use was via friends, acquaintances and/or family. Around 25% first heard of the substance

* Mean BMI 23.6 (standard deviation 3.6) kg/m^2.

through smart shops or pharmacies, and 17% first heard of it via the Internet.

All 304 respondents to the Internet questionnaire had used ephedra at some stage in their life (lifetime prevalence). Of these, 237 (78%) had used it in the year prior to completing the questionnaire and were designated as recent users. Of these recent users, 123 respondents (52%) had used ephedra in the month prior to participating in the study, and were designated as current users. Of the recent users, 55% usually used ephedra when alone, and about 25% usually used it when with friends.

Before the sale of ephedra was banned, the drug was marketed under various brand names. Each brand contained a different dosage and usually a variable quantity of additional substances, such as caffeine. Ephedra-based products from a pharmacy usually contained a lower quantity of the active ingredient than products from a smart shop. Over 60% of the respondents reported that they used one or two dosages per occasion, but the additional written comments showed that the dosage might differ according to the occasion. For example, a 27-year-old man reported that he took one tablet when he had to work, and two or three tablets when he was on a long night out. A woman of a similar age explained that she took one ephedra tablet before breakfast on a daily basis. She had used the drug over 50 times in the previous year, exclusively for the purpose of losing weight.

For analysis of the data, the population of recent ephedra users (n = 237) was divided into two equal groups – one with a high frequency of use (13 times per year or more) and one with a low frequency of use (1 to 12 times per year). In the group of high-frequency users, women are over-represented compared with men (63% and 37%, respectively; χ^2 = 11.825, df = 1, P < 0.01).

Table 4.1 shows the percentage of respondents who had used ephedra and other psychoactive substances at least once in their lifetime, during the past year (recent use) and during the past month (current use). Apart from ephedra, alcohol and cannabis were the other substances most frequently used (tobacco was not included in this question).

Comparison with national prevalence data (in the far right-hand column) shows that this sample of ephedra users (both male and female) were more experienced substance users than those aged 20–24 years in the whole Dutch population.

For further analyses, respondents were then categorised according to the types of drugs that they had used in the previous year. If they had used ecstasy, amphetamines, cocaine, gamma-hydroxybutyrate (GHB) or heroin at least once, they were designated as 'hard drug users.' Of those ephedra users who were high-frequency users, a significantly smaller number had used hard drugs compared with those who were

Table 4.1: Substance use among recent ephedra users ($n = 237$)

Substance	Lifetime (%)	Recent use (previous year) (%)	Current use (previous month) (%)	NDM, age 20–24 years* lifetime (%)
Ephedra	100	100	52	Not available
Alcohol	98	95	87	92
Cannabis	76	52	42	42
Ecstasy	53	37	20	14
Magic mushrooms	47	25	10	Not available
Amphetamines	43	24	10	10
Cocaine	37	20	10	9
Tranquillisers	38	21	11	Not available
Gammahydroxybutrate	17	8	3	Not available
Heroin	3	–	–	0.4

* *Source:* NDM, *National Drug Monitor. Annual Report 2004.*[13]

low-frequency users. In addition, in the year prior to the study, significantly fewer female than male ephedra users had used hard drugs (41% and 59%, respectively).

Reasons for using ephedra

In the subsample of hard drug users, a distinct consumption pattern emerged. Female ephedra users consumed ephedra more frequently than males, but used hard drugs less often, whereas male ephedra users consumed less ephedra than female users, but used hard drugs more often. These patterns of use can be explained by looking at the recent users' reasons for using ephedra.

Table 4.2 lists the eight pre-defined statements that the respondents could choose to indicate their reasons for using ephedra. 'Losing weight' and 'dancing' were the most frequently reported reasons, but these are also the two reasons that differed significantly between men and women (73% of female users cited losing weight as a reason for using ephedra, compared with 29% of male users). Those who rated 'It helps me to lose weight' as highly applicable to them were found to have a higher BMI than those who considered losing weight to be less applicable.* Over half of the men reported that they used ephedra to enable them to dance longer, compared with 37% of the women.

Women therefore use ephedra predominantly in order to lose weight. They also use the drug more frequently than do men. This suggests that

* BMI of those rating 'It helps me to lose weight' as highly applicable to them = 24.5 kg/m^2; BMI of those rating it as less applicable = 22.7 kg/m^2; $P < 0.01$.

Table 4.2: Reasons for using ephedra among recent users ($n = 237$)

I use(d) ephedra because:	Male* (n = 115) (%)	Female* (n = 122) (%)	Total* (n = 237) (%)
1 It helps me to lose weight†	29	73	52
2 I can dance for longer†	55	37	46
3 I like its 'high'	35	29	32
4 It enhances my athletic performance	29	34	31
5 It helps me to do my job	24	16	20
6 I can cope with the effect of alcohol better	19	11	15
7 It helps me when I feel down	10	11	11
8 It helps me to study	15	7	11

* Those who rated each statement as 4 or 5 on a scale where 1 = not at all applicable and 5 = highly applicable.
† Significant differences between male and female users where $P < 0.01$.

women use ephedra as a course of treatment to lose weight, as set out in the instructions on the packaging of many of the ephedra-containing dietary supplements, namely one or two tablets per day for a few weeks, followed by a 'rest period.'

Table 4.2 also shows that ephedra is used for a variety of reasons. A factor analysis (with varimax rotation) of motives reveals two components that explain 56% of the variance, namely pleasure (motives 2, 3 and 6) and performance (motives 1, 4, 5 and 7). However, the presence of 'losing weight' (motive 1) in the performance category seems out of place. Closer examination of the factor analysis (*see* Table 4.3) reveals that this item score (0.344) is considerably lower than that of the other items. This can probably be explained by the different nature of weight loss compared with the other two performance items. In the case of

Table 4.3: Reasons for using ephedra among recent users: factor analysis ($n = 237$)

I use(d) ephedra because:	Factor 1 (pleasure)	Factor 2 (performance)
1 It helps me to lose weight		0.344
2 I can dance for longer	0.779	
3 I like its 'high'	0.732	
4 It enhances my athletic performance		0.617
5 It helps me to do my job		0.790
6 I can cope with the effect of alcohol better	0.709	
7 It helps me when I feel down		0.705
8 It helps me to study		0.687
Explained variance	29.24	27.13

'pleasure' and 'dancing', the immediate energising effects of ephedra are central. However, weight loss is a secondary effect, resulting from suppression of appetite, usually combined with increased physical exercise.

Therefore, based on the interpretation of the factor analysis, three groups of ephedra users emerge, namely 'pleasure seekers', 'performers' and 'slimmers.' However, because many respondents indicated more than one reason for using ephedra, these groups are not exclusive.

Perceived effects, health problems and dependence

The reasons for using ephedra reflect the stimulant characteristics of the substance, and the same applies to its perceived effects. The respondents were presented with 13 pre-defined possible effects of ephedra, and were asked to indicate on a 5-point Likert scale the extent to which each applied to them. A factor analysis clustered the effects into three groups, namely mood/performance enhancement, (undesirable) side-effects and suppression of appetite. Together these account for 57% of the variance.

Of the recent ephedra users, almost 75% were aware that ephedra use may have negative health consequences, and 39 of these respondents (17%) reported that they had had health problems as a result of using ephedra (*see* Table 4.4).

Health problems associated with ephedra use were reported by 10% of the recent users, mainly women whose reason for using the substance was to lose weight. The finding that a larger proportion reported only having 'some experience' of health problems could be explained by respondents' caution when attributing these problems to ephedra use. They might be aware that health complaints can also result from an

Table 4.4: Recent ephedra users reporting health problems attributed to ephedra use (*n* = 237)

Health problem	Some experience* (%)	More experience† (%)	Total‡ (%)
Cardiac arrhythmia	6	4	9
Hypertension	9	2	10
Myocardial infarction	2	0	2
Stroke	2	0	2
Exhaustion	3	6	8
Underweight	4	1	5
Psychosis	5	1	6

* Those who rated their experience of each health problem as 2 or 3 on a scale where 1 = not at all applicable and 5 = highly applicable.
† Those who rated their experience of each health problem as 4 or 5 on a scale where 1 = not at all applicable and 5 = highly applicable.
‡ Rows do not add up to the exact total because the percentages have been rounded up or down.

interaction of ephedra with other factors, such as their lifestyle or pre-existing health problems.

Depression was not listed as a health effect in the questionnaire, but was reported by two people in the free-text boxes. For example, a 24-year-old male university student, who used ephedra exclusively for going out, described '*a light depression that, in my opinion, has been caused by using ephedra too often and too much, which has caused me to (temporarily) stop using ephedra.*'

The Internet questionnaire included three statements that may provide some insight into ephedra dependence.[14] Again using a 5-point Likert scale, where 1 = not at all applicable and 5 = highly applicable, 48% of the sample agreed that 'I have felt the need to use less ephedra' was applicable to them, 31% agreed that 'I find it difficult to stop using ephedra' and 16% agreed that 'I use ephedra to forget my worries.' Although the wording of these statements does not allow definitive conclusions to be drawn about whether or not the sample had dependency problems, the responses indicate that some respondents had to make an effort to control their ephedra use. Significantly more female than male users reported problems with controlling their use of ephedra (χ^2 = 10.743; df = 1; P < 0.01). Among those who used ephedra for slimming purposes, more reported problems with control compared with users for whom weight loss was less applicable (χ^2 = 4.075; df = 1; P < 0.05). This may reflect underlying problems with control over body weight.

Change in consumption patterns

Changes in consumption patterns that were attributed to the ban on ephedra were explored by asking recent ephedra users how applicable seven statements were to them (*see* Table 4.5). Three of these statements covered behaviour (1 to 3), three dealt with market conditions (4 to 6), and one covered attitude (7). Statements 4 to 7 were offered only to those who reported that they had reduced their ephedra use as a result of the ban. Table 4.5 shows the percentages of respondents who considered each statement to be very applicable to them.

Of the 237 recent ephedra users, 44% consumed the drug less often due to the ban, and 30% of them cited decreased availability as a reason for this (an increase in the price of ephedra may be interpreted as a decrease in availability to people who are financially less well off).

In the free-text boxes and during the face-to-face interviews the study participants reported that between the announcement of the ban and the actual start of the ban (a two-month period) they stocked up on ephedra. They then followed the strategy of gradually reducing their frequency of use so that their stock would last longer. Another reason for decreasing

Table 4.5: Recent ephedra users' change in consumption pattern attributed to the ban on ephedra (*n* = 237)

	% *
1 I use ephedra less often	44
2 I use less ephedra per occasion	20
3 I use ephedra more consciously	23
Have you used less ephedra for one of the following reasons? (*n* = 99†)	
4 Ephedra is harder to get	30
5 Ephedra has become more expensive	13
6 The quality of ephedra has worsened	6
7 I don't want to break the law	7

* Those who rated each statement as 4 or 5 on a scale where 1 = not at all applicable and 5 = highly applicable.
† This question was only presented to those who had reduced their use of ephedra since the ban.

ephedra use emerged from the face-to-face interviews. This was a change in attitude to its effects on health, prompted by the ban on its sales. Two of the interviewees perceived the ban as government confirmation of their suspicion that ephedra use was 'unhealthy' and therefore they should not use it. Nevertheless, both interviewees had purchased a considerable amount of ephedra when they heard of the forthcoming ban.

Substitutes for ephedra

When ephedra was still a legal product, smart shops marketed it as a herbal stimulant with fewer health risks than ecstasy or amphetamine. Indeed, some of the ephedra users remarked that they used the drug because it was legal and less dangerous than illegal stimulants. The question thus arises as to whether or not the ban on ephedra 'forced' ephedra users to (re)turn to the illegal drug market.

Of the recent ephedra users, 14% stated that since the ban they had used more illegal substances (ecstasy, amphetamines, cocaine, anabolic-like substances), or that they used them more often as a substitute for ephedra. Amphetamines and ecstasy were mentioned most frequently in this respect. In contrast, 27% of the recent users had used more legal substances (coffee, tobacco, cannabis), or used them more frequently, and half of them specified legal energisers or fat-burners as substitutes (usually dietary supplements based on caffeine or synefrine, marketed as 'ephedra-free' products). The questionnaire did not ask respondents to evaluate the effect of ephedra substitutes, but in the free-text box some respondents commented that the alternative dietary supplements were ineffective. As a 28-year-old male respondent, who had used both legal and illegal ephedra substitutes, stated:

> According to me there are no real equivalents [to ephedra]. The substitutes that work are just worse for your health (ecstasy, speed, coke), and the legal substitutes just don't work (I've tried them all, long before the ban).

Implications of the results

Most of the ephedra users in this self-selected sample were aged up to 30 years, and (among other reasons) ephedra was often used as a drug for 'pleasure' when going out to clubs. For the present study, pleasure in relation to ephedra was defined as being able to 'dance longer', to 'cope with alcohol effects' and to 'appreciate its high.' Some of the respondents used ephedra as part of a harm-reduction strategy, as they perceived it as a less dangerous drug than illegal stimulants. If ephedra is indeed used as a less harmful alternative to illegal stimulants, this group is likely to be very selective when choosing ephedra substitutes.

The demand for dietary supplements by those who want to lose weight is not likely to diminish in the coming years, and the group that used ephedra in order to lose weight was probably most affected by the ban on the drug in the Netherlands. The legal alternatives were considered to be ineffective by many of the respondents in this group. For example, synefrine (citrus aurantium) is available, but as yet it is unclear whether this substance can match the effects that are achieved with ephedra. Moreover, synefrine may increase cardiovascular risks, especially if it is used in combination with caffeine.[15] Unfortunately, in this study the group that appeared to need ephedra most to help them with their weight problems was also the group that reported the highest frequency of ephedra use. Consequently, they also experienced more undesirable side-effects and related health complaints, including problems with control over use. Central to weight loss is the balance between calorie intake and calories used, and apparently the use of ephedra (or similar substances) helps to achieve and maintain this balance. Although among the study's slimmers the average BMI (24.5 kg/m^2) is not alarming (a BMI over 25 kg/m^2 is deemed overweight[16]), these individuals should be informed about how to achieve and maintain a healthy energy balance. It is recommended, therefore, that on a national basis all dietary supplements should be accompanied by a leaflet giving information on a healthy lifestyle.

The effect of the ban itself may change attitudes towards ephedra, although this was only reported by two interviewees. It could be postulated that banning a substance has both a practical and a symbolic effect. It reduces availability, but it may also convince some potential users not to start or some current users to discontinue using it. Users and potential users may also be deterred by the health risks that legitimise the ban. To consider this further, it is necessary to make a distinction between use of ephedra for pleasure and for weight-loss purposes.

Seen from the perspective of use for pleasure, if an illegal substance offers clear (perceived) benefits to its consumers, it is likely that it will be widely used. Examples of this include ecstasy and cocaine, which among certain age groups have lifetime prevalence rates of up to 14%. However, ephedra-containing products (legal or illegal) never gained the popularity of cocaine or ecstasy, possibly because of their relatively modest effects. It is unlikely that individuals who used ephedra for pleasure were deterred by the ban, and reduced use of the drug was probably due to its limited availability.

Viewed from a weight-loss perspective, the ban on ephedra may have had both a practical effect (because of its limited availability) and a symbolic effect. If a substance has proved to be effective to the consumer, but also involves health risks, the pros and cons of its continued use will be carefully considered. Those who experience strong or unpleasant side-effects when they use ephedra may have their suspicions confirmed that ephedra is not as harmless as they previously thought. It is likely that in this group of ephedra users the ban also had a strong symbolic effect.

Conclusion

One year after the ban on ephedra it is unclear how the illicit market for this drug has developed and whether or not it will become part of the typical selection of illicit drugs (along with, for example, ecstasy and amphetamine) offered by dealers. Undoubtedly ephedra will remain available 'under the counter' in some smart shops, and the Internet will continue to play an important role in supply and demand. These developments should be monitored in order to assess the effect of the ephedra ban on drug-using patterns, the health problems of ephedra users, and the illegal drug market.

References

1 Shekelle PG, Hardy ML, Morton SC *et al*. Efficacy and safety of ephedra and ephedrine for weight loss and athletic performance: a meta-analysis. *JAMA*. 2003; **289**: 1537–45.

2 Ministry of Public Health, Welfare and Sport. *Smartshops en Nieuwe Trends in het Gebruik van Psycho-actieve Stoffen: Nota van de werkgroep Smart Shops [Smart Shops and New Trends in the Use of Psychoactive Substances: report of the working group Smart Shops]*. Rijswijk: Ministry of Public Health, Welfare and Sport; 1998.

3 Ephedra-alkaloïden verboden in levensmiddelen [Ephedra-alkaloids banned in foods]. *State Courant*, Internet edition, 6 February 2004.

4 Substances and classifications table. Legal reports: European legal database on drugs; http://eldd.emcdda.eu.int (accessed 31 August 2005).

5 Chan EL, Ahmed TM, Wang M *et al*. History of medicine and nephrology in Asia. *Am J Nephrol*. 1994; **14**: 295–301.

6 Powers ME. Ephedra and its application to sports performance: another concern for the athletic trainer? *J Athletic Training*. 2001; **26**: 420–24.

7 Abourashed EA, El-Alfy AT, Khan IA *et al*. Ephedra in perspective – a current review. *Phytother Res*. 2003; **17**: 703–12.

8 Bent S, Tiedt TN, Odden MC *et al*. The relative safety of ephedra compared with other herbal products. *Ann Intern Med*. 2003; **138**: 468–71.

9 Lenz TL, Hamilton WR. Supplemental products used for weight loss. *J Am Pharm Assoc*. 2004; **44**: 59–68.

10 Naik SD, Freudenberger RS. Ephedra-associated cardiomyopathy. *Ann Pharmacother*. 2004; **38**: 400–3.

11 Samenuk D, Link MS, Homoud MK *et al*. Adverse cardiovascular events temporally associated with ma huang, a herbal source of ephedrine. *Mayo Clin Proc*. 2002; **77**: 12–16.

12 Haller CA, Jacob P III, Benowitz NL. Pharmacology of ephedra alkaloids and caffeine after single-dose dietary supplement use. *Clin Pharmacol Ther*. 2002; **71**: 421–32.

13 Trimbos Institute. *National Drug Monitor. Annual Report 2004*. Utrecht: Trimbos Institute; 2004.

14 Cornel M, Knibbe RA, van Zutphen WM *et al*. Problem drinking in a general practice population: the construction of an interval scale for severity of problem drinking. *J Stud Alcohol*. 1994; **55**: 466–70.

15 Marcus DM, Grollman AP. Ephedra-free is not danger-free. *Science*. 2003; **301**: 1669–71.

16 World Health Organization. *Obesity and Overweight. Factsheet. Global strategy on diet, physical activity and health*; www.who.int/dietphysicalactivity/media/en/gsfs_obesity.pdf (accessed 15 March 2006).

Chapter 5

Khat and the creation of tradition in the Somali diaspora

Axel Klein

In the Somali community in the UK, few issues are as contentious as the status of khat. Many maintain that it lies at the root of the social and medical problems that trouble a significant proportion of the community. To others it is an innocent stimulant and an important aspect of their culture. However, opinion is unanimous that khat use is part of the Somali tradition, with long historical roots. This chapter argues that this is a misreading of history and that khat has only gained popularity among Somali users in recent decades. The problems associated with khat use are therefore not simply reducible to the pharmacological properties of the drug, but need to take into account a new cultural context of its use within the UK.

This chapter is based on a literature review and interviews with informants from Somali and Yemeni communities in London, Sheffield, Stockholm and Toronto. Interviews were conducted between December 2003 and June 2005 as part of an interdisciplinary research project entitled *The khat nexus: transnational consumption in a global economy*.[a]

Tradition and history

Somalis in Europe and North America are associated with the regular use of khat, a stimulant that among these countries is only legal in the UK and the Netherlands. This chapter will show how Somalis living in the UK are divided about the status of khat, some linking its use to problems such as unemployment, social exclusion, family breakdown and poor health. In contrast, many argue that khat is part of Somali tradition and culture. In fact, khat was not widely used in Somalia until the 1970s, and the subsequent ban, civil war and exile have all prevented the evolution of a culture of consumption with inbuilt harm-reducing customs and etiquette. Somalis are therefore vulnerable to problematic khat use.

The seminal collection of essays edited by the historians Hobsbawm and Ranger[1] is predicated on the claim that traditions do not have to be very old to be keenly appreciated as a core element in the identity of a nation, tribe or ethnic group. For example, the claim of Scottish clans that their customs date back for centuries is essential for their legitimacy and authenticity. In many cases, as in the purported link between tartan kilts and ancient highland clans, the line between myth and fiction is fluid. Although this may not matter when consolidating collective identity and facilitating group membership, it does have implications for managing the impact and consequences of such 'traditions.' This is particularly relevant when traditions revolve around the consumption of psychoactive substances, as in the case of khat among the Somali population. In other cultural contexts, enjoyment of a drug followed successful domestication, during which users learned to tame its powers. For example, the Ancient Greeks were terrified of alcohol until they learned from Dionysus to mix their wine with water.[2] The role of intermediaries, demi-gods or cultural heroes is often crucial in teaching people about controlled substance use, as for instance in the sacramental use of peyote among Native Americans.[3] In the case of khat, vernacular traditions in Yemen and Ethiopia[4] credit observant shepherds with the initial discovery of the shrub's stimulant properties. Interestingly, this 'myth of origin' is replicated in the new khat-growing areas of Uganda.[5]

For the Somali community in the UK, thousands of miles removed from the fields where the 'flowers of paradise'[4] bloom, the question of origin is of little pertinence. Exposure to the stricter Islamic schools that dominate British mosques may further discourage light-hearted references to apocryphal and possible pre-Islamic traditions. Important for the purpose of this chapter is the fact that within the community the chewing of khat, regardless of its origin, is widely recognised as a traditional custom linking current generations with their forefathers.

One of the arguments marshalled by informants in favour of khat, reported in the first research into Somali attitudes towards the drug, was that it helped to maintain cultural identity.[6] This idea that khat provides a link with Somalia is repeated in other research among UK Somalis, many of whom celebrate – or at least justify – khat in terms of culture and tradition.[7-9] According to a young Somali informant in Southall, London, 'khat is harmless, it's what they have always done back in Somalia.' Other Somalis have contrasted khat favourably with alcohol, compared the khat-chewing café (*mafrish*) to the pub,[10] and denied that khat is a 'drug.'[11] The Home Office does not regard the matter as quite so straightforward, and has commissioned successive research studies.[6-8] In 2005, the Home Secretary referred the question of khat's legal status to the Advisory Council on the Misuse of Drugs. After careful consideration of the evidence, the expert committee recommended in January 2006 that the status of khat should remain unchanged for the time being. It is possible that this decision will be revised in the process of the ongoing review of the drug classification mechanism.

Within the Somali community, opinions on khat are deeply divided. A large number of research study informants[7,8,12] are strongly in favour of a prohibition on khat import and distribution. Even some of the chewers themselves would like to see it banned,[9] although others insist that any ban should be completely effective, 'for if there was some around, I would find it.' Many proponents of a ban argue that it is not khat use per se that is the problem, but khat use in England, where the substance is allegedly stronger, more readily available, cheaper and taken in larger quantities than in Somalia. This contrast between culturally integrated traditional use and modern dysfunctional use is a familiar theme in the literature of drug and alcohol studies,[13] and has been employed by international drug control agencies as a central justification for the prohibition and eradication of plant-derived substances with ancient histories of medical, religious and cultural use.[14] In the case of Somalis, however, this representation is fundamentally misleading. Khat may be part of the culture, but it is not part of the history.

The Somali khat tradition

Khat (*Catha edulis*), also known as qat, chat and miraa, is a shrub that grows wild across much of Africa and Asia, favouring altitudes of between 5,000 and 6,500 feet above sea level. The oldest records show that khat was used in the highlands of Yemen and Ethiopia as early as the fourteenth century. It is also well established in the Meru mountains of Kenya. Somalia, by contrast, is an arid, low-lying country dominated by scrubland and savannah. In the pre-colonial era, the majority of the population were pastoralists, and there were pockets of intensive agricultural production in the river valleys and along the coast. Both as groups and individually, Somalis travelled widely and participated in the regional exchange economy, which was centred on the trade of meat, milk, leather and other animal products in exchange for vegetable produce. The trade between protein-producing lowlands, populated by nomadic groups, and the sedentary farmers of the highlands is a well-established feature in the Horn of Africa. Via this exchange system, Somalis were able to access agricultural produce that they could not grow in their own region. There was therefore a cultural memory and an awareness of exogenous crops such as khat.

In Somalia during this time, khat was only cultivated on small farms in the hill country in the north, also known as Somaliland.[b] For the most part, khat chewers depended upon imports from Harar in Ethiopia. As the camel was the only means of transporting goods, only the western fringes of Somaliland and Ogaden could obtain fresh khat. It was used for medical purposes and as an appetite suppressant, of particular value during long migratory treks,[15] but historically most Somalis would experience khat after the psychoactive compounds had decomposed. For the most part, however, Somalis had no experience of khat until the mid-twentieth century. Road construction in Ethiopia during the 1930s and 1940s opened up the khat-producing highlands of Harar to motor transport. As a result, khat became increasingly available in northern Somaliland, and quickly became more popular than the poorer-quality domestically grown plant.

Khat did not arrive in southern Somaliland and the capital of Mogadishu until the 1970s. At the time, khat chewing was widely perceived as a strange and foreign custom, popularised by returning migrant workers who had been exposed to the habit and who earned sufficient money to buy khat. The practice was quickly taken up by 'progressive' sections of the population, and developed into a pastime that for many came to typify Somali modernity – consumer-oriented, pleasure-seeking and supra-tribal.[16] Without a tradition of their own, Mogadishu khat chewers looked towards more established khat cultures. The very institution of the *mafrish* was borrowed from Yemen, and even the furniture, cushions to lie on, the accompanying tea and *sisha* water pipes were taken from the Yemeni model. In the first few years, musicians attending *mafrishes* would play songs from Somaliland, until those from the south had written their own.

The incipient khat consumer culture did not last long. In 1983, the authoritarian regime of Siyad Barre banned the importation and sale of khat. The official explanation was that khat was alien to Somali culture and was corrupting the public.[17] An eradication campaign was launched in northern Somalia, where crops were destroyed by troops, fanning the flames of a smouldering inter-regional conflict. Khat returned in a different guise following the overthrow of the Siyad Barre government in 1991, after which central authority in Somali disintegrated and the state collapsed. Different parts of the country came under the control of so-called warlords, who held on to their positions of power by employing militia forces. These consisted largely of young men, who were paid in bullets and in daily rations of khat imported by plane from Kenya. Even at the height of the Somali famine in the early 1990s, khat continued to be available and cargo space was given over to khat rather than to food imports.[18]

The image of the khat-crazed Somali gunslinger gained notoriety in the USA during the brief military intervention in Somalia to support the United Nations (UN) feeding programme. In order to help to pacify the country, the army tried to capture the warlord General Mohammed Farrah Aideed. In the failed attempt, two helicopters were shot down, several US servicemen and hundreds of Somalis were killed. Subsequently, the US authorities explained the debacle with reference to khat. One US website depicts a *mooryaan* (young warrior) holding an AK47 with the caption '*Khat eater waiting for a new target.*'[19] The substance was subsequently banned in the USA, where its importation and distribution are treated as serious offences.

Khat use in a global market

Within the last 30 years, the dramatic expansion of air cargo has made East African khat available in European and American markets. So far, most consumers in western countries originate from Eastern Africa and the Middle East. There is no evidence that khat use has been taken up by the mainstream population.[11] The lack of popularity outside the core immigrant groups is partly explained by the unfamiliar mode of administration. Shoots of khat are tied into bundles weighing 100–200 grams and wrapped in banana leaves to keep them fresh. The consumer picks off leaves and stems and chews these slowly into a quid that is stored in the side of the mouth. When all the juice has been extracted, the detritus is either swallowed or discarded.

The effect of khat is biphasic, beginning with vigorous stimulation of the central nervous system, resulting in animated behaviour and lively discussion. Then follows a tranquil, introspective phase, celebrated by poets and musicians for its inspirational powers.[20] In the UK, drug markets are already amply supplied with far more powerful stimulants, such as amphetamine and cocaine, and communal drug use is not only predominantly recreational, but also individualistic and hedonistic. There is little need for a drug with a culture of use that is mainly communal, reflective and even devotional.

Khat-chewing Somalis in the UK pursue their habit either in *mafrishes* (commercial premises where khat is sold and chewed) or in private homes. The available research testifies to the social dimension of khat use. People gather to chew, chat, drink soft drinks and smoke large quantities of tobacco. Indeed, some of the physical health problems associated with khat are caused by the cigarettes, water pipes and sugary drinks that accompany khat consumption.[21] Literature from the Yemen and Ethiopia highlights the importance of khat in relation to the working day and week.[11,21–25] It is used as a performance enhancer by farmers in the field, lorry drivers and students, and for relaxation by traders, craftsmen and office workers. This provides one possible indicator to the perceived problematic nature of khat use in the UK, where it is detached from the rhythm of working life, as unemployment among Somalis in the UK is rampant.

The invigorating qualities of khat derive from two alkaloids, identified as cathine and cathinone, which resemble amphetamine. However, they are highly unstable and disintegrate within 72 hours. Three days after harvest, khat is psychoactively ineffective and commercially worthless. Both cathine and cathinone are controlled substances in the UK, and their extraction is illegal.[c] However, the khat leaves can be imported legitimately as a vegetable. According to Her Majesty's Customs and Excise, an estimated 10,000 tons of khat pass through Heathrow airport annually, much of it destined for re-export. London, with good air links to Kenya, Yemen and Ethiopia, serves as a hub for global distribution. Given that khat is sold at £200 per kilo in the USA, compared with £10 in the UK, the incentives for export are obvious.

Campaigning against khat use

For the Somali activists campaigning for a ban on khat and their supporters within the UK, the British government's laissez-faire attitude is scandalous. As some see it, allowing khat to come into the UK in order to wreak havoc among the Somali community is seen as part of an insidious campaign against them. This is reinforced by the view that the British have formed opinions about khat use from their colonial experience in Somaliland and Aden. Colonial administrators in the 1950s associated the chewing of khat with the early nationalist protest movement in Somaliland,[16,24] and sought to prohibit its importation into Aden for mercantile reasons.[26] According to one informant, many Somali women compare the UK government's tolerance of khat with its harsh measures against cocaine and heroin, drugs with which few Somalis have become involved, but which are seen to present considerable difficulties for the white population. Women are prominent in the anti-khat campaign for a number of reasons. The Somali migration to the UK was often headed by women with their children. By the time their husbands arrived, the women had established themselves, learned the language and begun to negotiate their way around the system.[27] Once the men arrived, they found it difficult to reclaim their traditional authority, as they found it difficult to find work and act as providers. Many took to visiting the *mafrish*, diverting state benefit money to the purchase of khat. As a consequence, women have emerged as activists in the campaign to prohibit khat importation.

The difference between UK-based Somali complaints about khat and those of colonial administrators is telling. In the latter case, the objections were made on political and economic grounds. Users were more boisterous and assertive after chewing, whilst the imports from neighbouring Ethiopia were seen as an outflow of wealth from the British Empire. Contemporary campaigners and critics, by contrast, are concerned with the adverse impact of khat use on the well-being of the individual user, their family and the whole Somali community. At the forefront of these concerns are the claims that khat use leads to a range of mental health disorders, including hypnagogic hallucinations, mood swings, functional mood disorder, anxiety, sleeping disorders, loss of appetite and depression.[28–32] However, many commentators are cautious about making direct causal links between khat and the above conditions, because most studies have been conducted on small samples and have failed to control for possible confounding factors.[33] This is of particular importance in studies of immigrants, many of whom suffer from severe post-traumatic stress disorder after fleeing the violence of a civil war as well as famine, and experiencing the traumas of migration. Advocates for khat control have therefore sought to base their assertions on more solid ground. Khat, it is claimed, diverts active Somali men from the workplace, drains state-benefit-dependent household budgets, puts a strain on family relationships, and prevents the integration of Somalis into the UK mainstream.

Most importantly, perhaps, khat has become a proxy in a longstanding discussion about gender roles as Somalis in the UK renegotiate their social contracts as refugees-cum-citizens within a modern, multicultural country. According to one community leader, 'The women are going out to work, taking the children to school, doing the shopping, and the men are doing nothing but [khat] chewing.'[34] As campaigners have tapped into existing political mechanisms, policy makers are becoming involved with a very different slant on khat use and the call for 'action.' A member of the UK Parliament summarised the situation as follows:

> there are large numbers of people in west London who chew khat all night long, becoming increasingly aggressive, [then] come home in the morning, beat up the wife and try to sleep through the day.[35]

His colleague called upon the Home Secretary to control khat, as it was 'causing havoc in the Somali community.'[34]

The social context of khat use by Somalis in the UK

With the spotlight on the Somali community, little attention is being paid to the experience of other UK immigrant communities, particularly the Ethiopian and Yemeni communities, but the findings of two studies funded by the Home Office show clear divergences in the attitude of communities towards drugs. One study reports that 'Interviews with Ethiopian and Kenyan community members suggested that levels of khat use were not considered problematic'[7] and that most of the Yemeni men who were interviewed 'thought that khat was "not a drug", and therefore did not have the disadvantages of one.'[8] Ethiopian and Yemeni informants explained these attitudes by pointing out that Somalis chewed the drug for longer, not because of addiction but because they 'believed in it more', or because:

> while their [Yemeni] community had been in Britain for many years, including into a second generation, many Somalis were war refugees who had only been here for a few years, were more likely to be unemployed and to have 'nothing to do.'[8]

Such statements are shifting the focus away from khat and its pharmacological properties. Instead of approaching khat as a problem that is exacerbating the social and medical problems of the Somali community, they cite the traumatic personal histories and the difficulty in adjustment to the UK to explain the community's uneasy relationship with the substance. In their view, it is not khat that is the problem, but the surrounding circumstances of the users and of use. Known as 'set and setting', these are established principles in the sociology of drug use. The difficulties experienced by Somalis in the UK as a result of trauma, migration and continuing poverty and marginalisation in this country have also been emphasised by Somali researchers.[12,36]

Somehow, the claim that khat chewing forms an integral part of the Somali tradition remains unchallenged in the UK-based research exercises.[6–8,37] For the most part, researchers are content with the assertion that khat use in the UK is different to that in Somalia, and that khat in the UK is stronger, cheaper, more widely available or taken in a different context. Moreover, most qualitative research exercises have concentrated on collecting data on perceptions and attitudes towards khat among the Somali community. Researchers have rarely triangulated their findings on patterns of khat use with information on the culture, history and socio-economic conditions of its use in the Horn of Africa. This is part of an insularity that is perhaps typical of the drugs field, but critical when working with minority ethnic populations. However, when analysing the pathology of khat use by Somalis in the UK, an understanding of the historical background is pertinent.

Khat and the invention of tradition

Much of the discussion of khat has focused on its pharmacological properties and its association with medical conditions and social harm. While the community and researchers try to find ways of addressing the different pattern of khat use in the UK, it is the 'false memory' or creation of tradition that holds the key to many of the associated problems.

Somalis who identify khat as part of their culture do so without really understanding the historical origin of this consumption pattern. This chapter has shown that, for most, this did not exist until the 1970s. It is this very lack of tradition that has contributed to the much wider incidence of problematic khat use among Somalis than among Yemeni or Ethiopian chewers. The historical record shows clearly how in both these old centres of khat production an elaborate culture of consumption had developed.[22–24] This included etiquette for appropriate use, and restrictions against excess. Somali users, on the other hand, only gained regular access to khat in the dysfunctional setting of the civil war and the refugee camps. There is therefore no cultural memory of socially acceptable use of the substance among Somalis.

At the same time, as Hobsbawm and Ranger[1] have shown, the relatively recent arrival of a custom does not negate its cultural appropriation. Khat has become an emblem of Somali culture within a short space of time. Indeed, along the shifting khat frontier of East Africa, particularly in Kenya and Uganda, Somalis are popularly associated with khat chewing,[5] and in Nairobi they have taken over much of the khat export trade, not just to Somalia but also to London.[11] Once here, patterns of use change again. Research among the UK population of khat chewers suggests that the majority of regular users began this practice before coming to the UK.[7–9,12] Young people may be introduced to khat, or even use it in peer groups, but with the exception of alcohol, Somalis in the UK are beginning to show substance use patterns resembling those of their non-Somali peers.[38]

Nevertheless, many Somalis in the UK do regard khat chewing as part of their tradition and culture. Having been raised in the UK, their information about Somalia is part of an oral tradition passed on by the elders. Many of them are avid chewers of khat and regular visitors to the *mafrish*. It is easy to see how a relatively recent phenomenon can be perceived as a traditional custom practised by one's forefathers. In reality it is but a recent trend, and the conventions and customs necessary to render it socially acceptable have yet to emerge. In the mean time, all of the parties involved in the debate on khat could benefit from a realistic reassessment of the history of khat use within Somali culture.

Endnotes

a This project was funded by the Economic and Social Science Research Council in the *Cultures of Consumption* series, grant number RES-143-25-0046. All informant citations, unless otherwise referenced, are taken from field notes collected as part of this project.

b This territory became a British protectorate. Like many African ethnic groups, the Somalis were split up among different European imperial rivals in the late-nineteenth-century 'Scramble for Africa.' The bulk of modern-day Somalia was colonised by

Italy, France incorporated a slither into its colony of Djibouti, and a southern part was absorbed into British Kenya. Even Ethiopia, the only African state to survive the colonial onslaught, took part by occupying the Ogaden.

c Cathine was found to be about half as potent as amphetamine and was added to schedule III, and cathinone was found to be about seven to ten times less potent and was added to schedule I of the UN Convention on Psychotropic Substances (1971) in 1986.

References

1 Hobsbawm E, Ranger T, editors. *The Invention of Tradition.* Cambridge: Cambridge University Press; 1983.
2 Escohotado A. *A Brief History of Drugs. From the Stone Age to the Stoned Age.* New York: Park Street Press; 1999.
3 French LA. *Addictions and Native Americans.* Westport, CT: Praeger; 2000.
4 Rushby K. *Eating the Flowers of Paradise: a journey through the drug fields of Ethiopia and Yemen.* London: Constable; 1998.
5 Beckerleg S. What harm? Kenyan and Ugandan perspectives on khat use. *African Affairs.* 2006; **105**: 219–41.
6 Griffiths P. *Qat Use in London: a study of qat use among a sample of Somalis living in London.* London: Home Office Drug Prevention Initiative; 1998.
7 Patel S, Wright S, Gammampila A. *Khat Use Among Somalis in Four English Cities.* London: Home Office; 2005.
8 Turning Point. *Khat Use in Somali, Ethiopian and Yemenin Communities in England: issues and solution.* London: Turning Point; 2005.
9 Woods D. *Khat Chewing and the Mental Health of Adult Somalis in Sheffield.* Sheffield: Somali Mental Health Project; 2005.
10 Klein A, Beckerleg S. Building castles of spit. In: Goodman J, Lovejoy P, Sherrat A, editors. *Consuming Habits: drugs in history and anthropology.* London: Routledge; 2006.
11 Anderson D, Beckerleg S, Hailu D *et al. The Khat Controversy: stimulating the debate on drugs.* Oxford: Berg; 2006.
12 Fowzi W. *Patterns of Khat Use Among Somalis in Camden.* London: Camden Drug and Alcohol Team; 2005.
13 Willis J. *Potent Brews: a social history of alcohol in East Africa, 1850–1999.* London: James Currey; 2002.
14 United Nations Drug Control Programme (UNDCP). *World Drug Report.* Vienna: UNDCP; 1997.
15 Lewis I. *A Modern History of the Somali.* London: James Currey; 2002.
16 Cassanelli L. Quat: a quasi-legal commodity. In: Appadurai A, editor. *The Social Life of Things: commodities in cultural perspective.* Cambridge: Cambridge University Press; 1986.
17 Ministry of Information and National Guidance. *Why was Khat Prohibited in Somalia?* Mogadishu: Ministry of Information and National Guidance; 1983.
18 Drysdale L. *Whatever Happened to Somalia? A tale of tragic blunders.* London: Haan; 1994.
19 www.borderpatrol.com/borderframe901.htm (accessed 26 March 2005).
20 Varisco D. On the meaning of chewing: the significance of qat (*Catha edulis*) in the Yemen-Arab-Republic. *Int J Middle East Stud.* 1986; **1**: 1–13.
21 Salam S. *Assessment of khat use amongst Yemeni khat chewers in Sheffield and Birmingham.* Unpublished MSc thesis. London: Queen Mary College; 2004.

22 Gebissa E. *Leaf of Allah: khat and agricultural transformation in Harerge, Ethiopia, 1875–1991*. Oxford: James Currey; 2003.

23 Kennedy J. *The Flower of Paradise: the institutionalized use of the drug qat in North Yemen*. Dordrecht: Kluwer/Reidel; 1987.

24 Krikorian A. Khat and its use: an historical perspective. In: *The Health and Socio-Economic Aspects of Khat Use*. Lausanne: International Council on Alcohol and Addictions; 1983.

25 Weir S. *Qat in Yemen: consumption and social change*. London: British Museum; 1985.

26 Brooks C. Khat: its production and trade in the Middle East. *Geogr J*. 1960; **126**: 52–9.

27 Harris H. *The Somali Community in the UK. What we know and how we know it*. London: Information Centre about Asylum and Refugees in the UK; 2004.

28 Granek M, Shalev A, Weingarten A. Khat-induced hypnagogic hallucinations. *Acta Psychiatr Scand*. 1988; **78**: 458–61.

29 Odenwald M, Nener F, Schauer M *et al*. Khat use as risk factor for psychotic disorder: a cross-sectional and case–control study in Somalia. *BioMedCentral Med*. 2005; **3**: 5.

30 Stefan J, Mathew. Khat chewing: an emerging drug concern. *Aust N Z J Psychiatry*. 2005; **39**: 322–6.

31 Pantelis C, Hindler C, Taylor J. Use and abuse of khat (*Catha edulis*): a review of the distribution, pharmacology and side-effects and a description of psychosis attributed to khat chewing. *Psychol Med*. 1989; **19**: 657–68.

32 Yousef G, Huq Z, Lambert T. Khat chewing as a cause of psychosis. *Br J Hosp Med*. 1995; **54**: 322–6.

33 Warfa N, Bhui K, Craig T. Post-migration geographical mobility, mental health and health service utilization among Somali refugees in the UK: a qualitative survey. *Health Place*. 2006; **12**(4): 503–15.

34 Summers C. Harmless habit or dangerous drug? *BBC News*, 5 January 2006.

35 *Hansard*, 18 January 2005.

36 Warfa N, Klein A, Bui K *et al*. Khat use and mental disorder. Unpublished.

37 Bashford J, Buffin J, Patel K. *Community Engagement. Report 2: the findings*. Preston: University of Central Lancashire, Centre for Ethnicity and Health; 2003.

38 Klein A. *Khat in Streatham: formulating a community response*. London: DrugScope; 2005.

Chapter 6

Characteristics of life in exile: vulnerability factors for substance use

Marjolein Muys

The aim of this chapter is to provide a theoretical understanding of the nature and extent of substance use among refugees. A theoretical model of self-medication is constructed and illustrated by means of data obtained from empirical research among refugees. The subjects of this chapter are those who have fled their home countries and applied for asylum in another country (asylum seekers), and those who have been granted asylum (refugees). Throughout, the term 'refugees' is used unless only asylum seekers are being discussed. The chapter contains a review of existing empirical studies of asylum seekers and refugees in Europe, North America and Australia. The empirical data are presented in order to illustrate a theoretical model that aims to provide a basis for future empirical studies.

Because many aspects of life in exile are associated with stress (for example, experiences of war in their home country, lack of privacy in asylum seekers' centres, adaptation to new situations, and boredom), the theoretical model of this study departs from the stress experience. 'Stress' is studied from the perspective of the conservation of resources (COR) theory, which has been presented by Hobfoll[1,2] as a general theory for understanding the nature and influence of stress. First the theoretical model is outlined, and then it is applied to life in exile. The general theoretical model departs from resource loss as a stress-inducing event. Because refugees experience an array of resource losses in all domains, it is argued that they lead a stressful life. Due to pre- and post-migration resource losses, poor mental health is expected. The next section uses empirical data to illustrate the fact that many refugees suffer from psychiatric disorders, and discusses why refugees are at high risk of adopting passive–avoidant strategies in order to cope with stress and poor mental health. The final section argues that because refugees have few resources in their host country, little control over their new situation and/or few personal resources (such as self-esteem), they are vulnerable to the problematic use of alcohol, prescription medication and illegal drugs.

It should be emphasised that the focus of this chapter on the vulnerability factors associated with living in exile does not detract from the remarkable resilience that is shown by many refugees.

Conservation of resources (COR) theory

COR theory is based on the premise that individuals strive to obtain, retain and protect that which they value – their 'resources.' These are the objects, conditions, personal characteristics and energies that are valued for survival, either directly or indirectly, or that serve as a means of achieving these resources:

> internal and external characteristics that individuals maintain and accumulate in service of having coping options and adjusting well.[1–4]

Loss of resources

In the COR model of stress, losses or gains of resources are the units of analysis. Stress will ensue under any of three conditions:

1 when there is threat of significant resource loss
2 when there is actual resource loss
3 when resources are invested without resulting in significant resource gain.

Resource loss can be acute or chronic. Acute resource loss is likely to result in stress because it is very rapid and the resource reservoir is emptied in the short term. Chronic resource loss exhausts all available resources to the extent that the entire resource reservoir can be emptied in the long term.[4]

COR theory posits that resource loss is central to the stress experience because it has a negative emotional impact. Exposure to stressful life events may have (long-lasting) implications for mental health.[5,6] Furthermore, resource loss cycles into further resource loss.[7]

Loss cycles

In order to deal with stress, people develop coping strategies, which have been defined as 'behaviours that are enacted to respond to recovery demands'.[8] COR theory postulates that additional resources must be invested in order to cope with previous resource loss.[9]

Two clusters of coping strategies can be distinguished, namely active–approach and passive–avoidant strategies. Active–approach coping strategies are directly aimed at changing the environment – the coping efforts actively address the stressor itself. Passive–avoidant coping strategies attempt to evade thoughts and feelings associated with the stressor.[5,8] The strategy adopted depends on the level of resources available to the individual, the extent to which the stressor can be controlled and/or the personal characteristics of the individual.

People with few resources are more likely to develop avoidance coping strategies, as they lack resources that could be invested in approach strategies. This implies that the fewer resources an individuals has, the more likely they are to be overwhelmed by the (threats of) losses they encounter, and coping efforts may therefore induce loss spirals among individuals with minimal resources. For example, an individual may engage in avoidance coping in order to prevent the loss of self-esteem that would result from focusing on the problem. This strategy may induce further loss, as the individual fails to address problems in their environment.[1,10]

The nature of the coping strategy that will be applied depends on the controllability of the stressor – that is, the degree to which stress can be mitigated or eliminated by an appropriate response.[11] Passive–avoidant coping strategies that address the emotions that accompany stress are likely to be applied when the stressor is outside the individual's control, and will be continued for as long as the stressor must be endured, or until a solution is possible. Individuals who are unable to control the source of stress and its solution are likely to adopt passive–avoidant strategies.

In addition to characteristics such as age, gender and previous exposure to stress, the reaction to stress is also shaped by internal or personal resources. Most important in this respect are aspects of self-esteem, linked to a sense of ability to successfully control and impact upon one's environment, especially in challenging circumstances.[5,6,9]

Substance use

The self-medication hypothesis postulates that substances are used as a means of achieving relief from symptoms of pre-existing stress and stress-related psychiatric disorders. Based on COR theory, it will be argued that there is a pathway from stress to substance use. Because people who experience great resource loss suffer from personal distress, those with few resources and low self-esteem who find themselves in uncontrollable situations will apply passive–avoidant coping strategies. Substance use is a typical example of passive–avoidant coping, as this strategy is a relatively easy way to cope with problems. Although minimal substance use (of illicit drugs, of prescription drugs obtained either via a doctor or illicitly, or of alcohol) may aid individuals during initial periods of distress, prolonged use of large amounts can lead to problematic use.[12]

Resource loss among refugees

There is often a multitude of loss experiences among refugees. In this section, it is argued that they may experience acute as well as chronic resource loss. Traumatic experiences in their home country may have induced acute loss, and refugees experience chronic loss if their resource reservoirs are not refilled in the host country.

Acute level: pre-migration trauma

From the perspective of COR theory, trauma can be characterised as acute loss, as it is rapid and extensive, and it results in rapid resource depletion. The individual is overwhelmed by the extent of what is lost, as traumatic loss affects all resource domains and leaves all resource reservoirs empty.[13,14]

Worldwide, many refugees have experienced severe trauma in their home countries. Table 6.1 provides an overview of the nature and prevalence of trauma exposure among refugees as demonstrated by empirical research and shows that data on refugee trauma are often conflicting and difficult to interpret because a variety of methods and instruments have been used for data collection, analyses and reporting.[15–30] In addition, the different kinds of trauma that refugees experience are diverse, and the prevalence rates for these traumas are equally diverse, even when similar ethnic groups are studied in similar settings.

Chronic level: post-migration loss

Resettlement stressors may be labelled as chronic stressors, since the conditions reported by refugees have a long duration. When people are bombarded by a series of ongoing stressful life events, COR theory suggests that, as resources are chronically threatened or depleted by their living conditions, coping options can be reduced and psychological distress may result.[1,31] The great losses suffered by refugees, discussed below, are those of cultural resources, the family, social status and future perspectives.

Refugees are usually confronted with a radically different environment in their host country. They face a new culture with a different social structure and specific social demands. This confrontation may cause

Table 6.1: Empirical data on the nature and prevalence of trauma exposure among refugees*

Reference	Country of origin	Host country	Setting†	Number of participants	Instruments‡	Being close to death	Forced isolation	Refugee camp	Imprisonment	Lack of food or water	Lack of shelter	Murder of family members or friends	Forced separation from family members	Torture	War, combat situation	Witnessed murder
16	Various	Norway	COS	240	HTQ	81%			36%				74%	15%	74%	33%
17	Iraq	UK	CLS	84	HTQ STAR					38%				65%		
18	Vietnam	Australia	COS	1,161	HTQ	14%	2%		13%	20%	3%	3%	11%	1%	6%	8%
19	SE Asia	USA	CLS	91	HTQ	60%	60%		37%	80%	70%		70%	50%	60%	
20,21	Various	Australia	ASC	40	HTQ	45%			16%	33%			42%	26%	50%	29%
22	Kosovo	UK	ASC	842	WTQ	88%				70%		58%				42%
23	Cambodia	USA	COS	50	PTI	80%		100%		80%		80%				
24	Bosnia	USA	CLS	20	CTEI			100%		100%		100%	100%			
25	SE Asia	USA	COS	129	CTEI		79%	92%		85%	82%	59%	81%			20%
26	Indochina	USA	CLS	52	LESHQ									100%		
27	Vietnam	USA	CLS	201		7%			5%					5%	3%	
28	Turkey Iran	Netherlands	COS	156			15%		83%			59%		59%	46%	7%
29	Cambodia	USA	COS	124	WTS			95%		85%	62%	85%	60%	21%		
30	Various	Sweden	CLS	149			5%		9%					70%	6%	10%

* Percentage values in italics are those from papers that did not give exact percentages.
† CLS, clinical setting; COS, community study; ASC, study in an asylum seekers' centre.
‡ HTQ, Harvard Trauma Questionnaire; STAR, Survivor of Torture Assessment Record; WTQ, War Trauma Questionnaire; PTI, Post-Traumatic Inventory; CTEI, Communal Traumatic Experiences Inventory; LESHQ, Life Events and Social History Questionnaire; WTS, War Trauma Scale.

feelings of not belonging, as familiar behaviour is no longer effective and social roles need to be played in a different manner. Such feelings of not belonging are associated with depression, and may be suppressed by substance use.[32-34] Every individual who faces a new environment will to some extent try to adapt to it. During this process, known as acculturation, individuals and groups undergo mutual changes when they come into contact with other cultures, and each culture influences the other. Refugees may therefore lose their traditional ways of living and suffer from acculturation stress.[35,36]

Many refugees are separated from their family and are stressed by worrying and thinking about the family members whom they left behind.[21] In the case of separation from a spouse and/or children, psychiatric disorders may occur.[37] Loss of family members in the sense of their death or disappearance is also associated with mental health problems.[29,38]

Despite persecution and danger in the country of origin, many refugees had a certain rank there that carried responsibilities and advantages, but in the host country, social position and social roles remain unclear, especially while refugees are waiting for a decision on asylum applications. This loss of prestige may cause depression.[32,39]

Loss of important life projects, such as a home that was built as a legacy to be passed on to the next generation, a business, or an anticipated retirement after a lifetime of employment are salient sources of distress for refugees. Because of these losses of acquired resources and a perspective on the future, many have become dependent on others and on social welfare in their host country.[40]

Mental health of refugees

Table 6.2 presents an overview of empirical data on the prevalence of psychiatric disorders (post-traumatic stress disorder, depression and anxiety) among refugees studied in clinical and community settings. The table reveals disparate findings. Several factors may in part account for these differences – for example, the time elapsed since the trauma, methods of sampling and measurement, and ethno-cultural differences in psychological responses. It is also possible that the significance and meanings underlying trauma experiences are more important than the detail of discrete events in determining risk of mental health problems. The discrepancies within the empirical data may be due to the non-applicability of western criteria to non-western cultures. Emotional distress experienced by members of a non-western culture may not be expressed in the same manner as that experienced by individuals in western countries.[41]

Table 6.2: Prevalence of mental disorders among refugees

Reference	Country of origin	Host country	Length of stay	Setting*	N	Instrument†	PTSD‡	Depression	Anxiety
16	Various	Norway	3 years	COS	240	HTQ	15%		
17	Iraq	UK		CLS	84	PSE, DSM-II-R, HTQ	11%		
21	Various	Australia	Mean = 3 years	ASC	40	CIDI, HSCL-25	37%	33%	25%
22	Kosovo	UK		ASC	120	CAPS, DSM-IV	39%	16%	
23	Cambodia	USA	4–6 years	COS	50	PTSD Checklist	86%	80%	
24	Bosnia	USA	Newcomers	CLS	20	PTSD Scale	65%	35%	
25	Kosovo	USA	Newcomers	COS	129	PDS	60%		
26	Indochina	USA		CLS	52	LESHQ, DIS	50%		
27	Vietnam	USA		CLS	201	SCID, ADIS-PTSD	3%	5.5%	3%
29	Cambodia	USA	Mean = 8 years	COS	124	DIS, DICA-R	45%	51%	
30	Various	Sweden	No data available	CLS	149	PTSD-I	83%		
36	Former Yugoslavia	Sweden	Newcomers + 3 years later	CLS	27	SCL-90-R, PSE	63%		
37	Vietnam	Norway	T1: 3 months T2: 3 years	COS	145		T1: 9% T2: 4%	T2: 18%	T2: 2%
38	Bosnia	Australia	More than 3 years	COS	126	CAPS	63%		
42	Bosnia	Sweden	3–4 years	COS	163	HSCL-25	28%	94%	97%
43	Bosnia	Sweden		ASC	206	PTSS-10	33%		
44	SE Asia	Canada	T1: new T2: 2 years T3: 10 years	COS	T1: 1,348 T2: 1,169 T3: 674	RPPSI Symptom Inventory		T1: 6% T2: 4% T3: 2%	

* CLS = clinical setting; COS = community study; ASC = study in an asylum seekers' centre; DSM-II-R = Diagnostic and Statistical Manual II Revisited; DSM-IV = Diagnostic and Statistical Manual IV; SCID = The Structured Clinical Interview for DSM-IV (SCID); ADIS-PTSD = Anxiety Disorders Interview Schedule Revised for Post Traumatic Stress Disorder; RPPSI = Refugee Resettlement Project Symptom Inventory.

† HTQ, Harvard Trauma Questionnaire; PSE, Present State Examination; DSM-II-R, Diagnostic and Statistical Manual II Revisited; CIDI, Composite International Diagnostic Interview; HSCL-25, Hopkins Symptom Checklist-25; CAPS, Clinician-Administered PTSD Scale; DSM-IV, Diagnostic and Statistical Manual IV; PDS, Post-traumatic Diagnostic Scale; LESHQ, Life Events and Social History Questionnaire; DIS, Diagnostic Interview Schedule; SCID, The Structured Clinical Interview for DSM-IV (SCID); ADIS-PTSD, Anxiety Disorders Interview Schedule Revised for Post Traumatic Stress Disorder; DICA–R, Diagnostic Interview for Children and Adolescents – Revised; SCL-90-R, Symptom Checklist-90-Revised; PTSS-10, Post-Traumatic Symptom Scale; RPPSI = Refugee Resettlement Project Symptom Inventory.

‡ PTSD, post-traumatic stress disorder.

Predictors of passive coping among refugees

As discussed earlier in this chapter, individuals who have few resources, who find themselves in stressful situations that they cannot control and/ or who have low self-esteem are likely to adopt passive–avoidant coping strategies.

Few resources

Because of the long-lasting difficulties in the host country, coping resources become overextended, resulting in destructive cycles of continued loss. Refugees have few resources to counter the loss of resources due to migration, and the scarcity of coping resources includes a lack of social resources, as well as language barriers, unemployment and poverty.

Social resources (particularly social support) are related to better emotional outcomes in the face of stress.[9] Refugees have a low level of social support, and this is associated with mental health problems.[16,17,21,36,37,42,45] However, social isolation might be the consequence of an individual's poor mental health, and not only its antecedent, as in many cases traumatised individuals tend to isolate themselves from others. Negative social conditions, which imply an unfavourable situation for mourning over traumatic losses, have a negative impact on the mental health of many refugees, and as a result post-traumatic stress disorder symptoms persist.[16,36,37]

Many refugees are unable to speak the language of their host country, even ten years after resettlement.[44] This causes stress[29,38] and makes it difficult to extend social networks to members of the host population.[16]

Unemployment rates among refugees are high,[16,21,46] and unemployment is known to be stressful.[16,17] Asylum seekers experience stress because they are not allowed to work, and refugees experience it because they are unable to find work.[21] The consequent loss of meaningful structure and activity in daily life is associated with mental health problems.[21]

Several empirical studies have examined the prevalence and impact on mental health of poverty, defined as 'not having enough money', 'financial problems', 'economic difficulties' and 'high dependence on social welfare.'[17,21,29,36,40,42] These studies show that insufficient income for safe and adequate housing and other basic necessities is a common source of stress among refugees.

Lack of control

Asylum seekers are typically concerned about a lack of control over their lives. For instance, many of them report frustration that an asylum seekers' centre takes care of all aspects of their lives (e.g. food supply, parenting, education, medical care, personal hygiene).[47] These frustrations and a lack of future perspective because of the unknown outcome of the asylum application render asylum seekers vulnerable to excessive use of alcohol, tobacco and other drugs.[48,49]

Low self-esteem

As was noted earlier, the self-esteem of refugees is affected by feelings of not belonging in the host country, and this can be exacerbated by experiences of racism. Approximately a quarter of studied samples of refugees have reported experiences of racism and discrimination.[17,45,50] These feelings and experiences hinder their attempts to see themselves as fulfilled and legitimate members of the host society.[32,47]

Substance use

The few studies that have investigated the use of alcohol, prescription medication and illegal drugs among refugees support the self-medication hypothesis – that substances are used to relieve symptoms of stress and mental ill health. Moreover, refugees are exposed to some risk factors that make them vulnerable to substance use, although some protective factors also exist.

Self-medication hypothesis

Dupont et al.[49] postulated that asylum seekers and refugees use substances in order to 'kill time', which suggests a functional pattern of use in relation to their past, present and future. Substance use may be related to past trauma in the country of origin, or to the eradication of memories of trauma before emigration. In the present, it may be related to the asylum-seeking process, with its long waiting periods, severe restrictions, insecurity and boredom. Substance use is also correlated with uncertainty about the future while waiting for the official decision on refugee status. Other studies on substance use among refugees support the self-medication hypothesis.[51–54]

Thus refugees are vulnerable to substance use, because this coping strategy enables them to self-medicate mental health problems that originate from pre- and/or post-migration loss. Because they have few resources with which to offset loss, little control over the situation in which they find themselves and/or low self-esteem, it is predicted that they may apply this passive–avoidant coping strategy.

Risk factors

The most significant risk factor for substance use in the host country is prior consumption in the home country. Refugees may use substances that are traditionally consumed by their ethnic or national group. The kind of substance refugees prefer, is, to a certain degree, connected to their country of origin and is influenced by the lifestyle, the cultural convictions and the values of the ethnic group.

Refugees may not only continue the patterns of substance use they brought with them from their home countries, but they may intensify them (e.g. khat use amongst Somalis in England, where the substance is taken in larger amounts than in Somalia; *see* Chapter 5). Restrictions on traditionally used substances in their home country may no longer apply in the country of resettlement: the self-medication motive may lead to the use of substances in larger amounts than the usual quantities consumed.[52,53]

Many refugees originate from countries without the traditions of alcohol or cannabis use found in the west.[53] The perceived permissive socio-cultural norms in the host country concerning the use of, particularly, these two substances, render new immigrants vulnerable to their use. During the acculturation process, refugees may adapt to patterns of substance use that are culturally accepted in the host country,[49,51,52] especially where some substances are widely available. Those who originate from cultures in which substance use is taboo are not acquainted with the risks and have not been educated to deal with them, and are also vulnerable to use escalating to a problematic level.

Protective factors

Despite the vulnerability of many refugees to substance use, several protective factors need to be taken into account. First, they may not want to jeopardise their residence permit by risking being discovered using drugs, and asylum seekers may not use drugs because they want to be considered 'good citizens' in order to obtain a residence permit. Secondly, those who acculturate less, and maintain a protective cultural identity[55] according to which substance use should be rejected, are at lower risk of substance use. A third protective factor exists if refugees follow a religion.[55] Many of the refugees interviewed by Fountain[51] cited their religion as a reason for not using drugs, and among Muslims the prohibition of alcohol has a protective effect on those who are devout.[56] Fourthly, some social factors protect against drug use, such as inclusion in peer groups, positive social contacts, and lasting relationships with people from the home country and new relationships forged with members of the host country's population.[55,56]

Conclusion

Using empirical data, this chapter has demonstrated that many refugees suffer from pre-migration and post-migration losses. Many have suffered severe trauma in their home country, including solitary confinement, imprisonment, torture, the murder of their families and friends, and war. In their host country, refugees suffer from the additional losses of cultural resources, loved ones and the extended family, social status and future perspectives. Based on COR theory, which emphasises the significance of resource loss, it has been shown that refugees are therefore subject to major stress.

In order to deal with stress and its negative impact on mental health, coping strategies are developed. However, the nature of these strategies (active–approach vs. passive–avoidant) will depend on the individual's situation and personal characteristics. Based on three characteristics (few resources, low controllability and/or low self-esteem) of life in exile, this chapter has argued that refugees are vulnerable to adopting passive–avoidant coping strategies because they have few resources at their disposal to counter the loss of resources. Consistent with the self-medication hypothesis, it has been argued that substance use is a plausible example of a passive–avoidant coping strategy.

In order to clarify the situation with regard to substance use among refugees, a better understanding of how and why refugees adopt coping strategies is needed.[54] The author is currently empirically testing the relative importance of the different elements of the theoretical model in the evolution of patterns of substance use. These elements will be studied in a multidimensional model that accounts for pre-migration trauma, post-migration stress, adaptation to patterns of use in the host country (acculturation), intensification of patterns of use from the home country, and the availability of substances in the host country. The relative importance of these elements in determining refugees' adoption of substance use as a coping strategy will be addressed. The general theoretical model will be tested by means of a case study of Iranian asylum seekers in Belgium. Because of their particularly stressful status compared with refugees, only asylum seekers and those without a residence permit will be interviewed. The aim of the study is to identify the most important factors that influence the evolution of patterns of substance use, and to examine the impact of those factors. On a theoretical level, the relative importance of these factors will be clarified in order to identify the most important risk factors for substance use among all refugees.

References

1 Hobfoll SE. Conservation of resources: a new attempt at conceptualising stress. *Am Psychol.* 1989; **44**: 513–24.

2 Hobfoll SE. *Stress, Culture and Community: the psychology and philosophy of stress.* New York: Plenum Press; 1998.

3 Hobfoll SE. Social and psychological resources and adaptation. *Rev Gen Psychol.* 2002; **6**: 307–24.

4 Hobfoll SE, Lilly RS. Resource conservation as a strategy for community psychology. *J Commun Psychol.* 1993; **21**: 128–48.

5 Holohan CJ, Moos RH. Life stress and health: personality, coping and family support in stress resistance. *J Pers Soc Psychol.* 1985; **49**: 739–47.

6 King LA, King DW, Keane TM *et al.* Resilience-recovery factors in post-traumatic stress disorder among female and male Vietnam veterans: hardiness, post-war social support and additional stressful life events. *J Pers Soc Psychol.* 1998; **74**: 420–34.

7 Bansal A, Monnier J, Hobfoll SE *et al.* Comparing men's and women's loss of perceived social and work resources following psychological distress. *J Soc Pers Relationships.* 2000; **17**: 265–81.

8 Benight CC, Ironson G, Klebe K *et al.* Conservation of resources and coping self-efficacy following a natural disaster: a causal model analysis where the environment meets the mind. *Anxiety Stress Coping.* 1999; **12**: 107–26.

9 Hobfoll SE, Johnson RJ, Ennis N *et al.* Resource loss, resource gain and emotional outcomes among inner-city women. *J Pers Soc Psychol.* 2003; **84**: 632–43.

10 Benotsch EG, Brailey K, Vasterling JJ *et al.* War zone stress, personal and environmental resources, and PTSD symptoms in Gulf War veterans: a longitudinal perspective. *J Abnorm Psychol.* 2000; **109**: 205–13.

11 Anisman H, Merali Z. Understanding stress: characteristics and caveats. *Alcohol Res Health.* 1999; **23**: 241–9.

12 Hobfoll SE, Spielberger CD, Breznitz FC *et al.* War-related stress. Addressing the stress of war and other traumatic events. *Am Psychol.* 1991; **46**: 848–55.

13 Hobfoll SE, Dunahoo CA, Monnier J. Conservation of resources and traumatic stress. In: Freedy JR, Hobfoll SE, editors. *Traumatic Stress: from theory to practice.* New York: Plenum Press; 1995.

14 Freedy JR, Hobfoll SE, Ribbe DP. Life events and adjustment: lessons for the Middle East. *Anxiety Stress Coping.* 1994; **7**: 191–203.

15 Hollifield M, Eckert V, Warner TD *et al.* Development of an inventory for measuring war-related events in refugees. *Compr Psychiatry.* 2002; **46**: 67–80.

16 Lie B. A 3-year follow-up study of psychosocial functioning and general symptoms in settled refugees. *Acta Psychiatr Scand.* 2002; **106**: 415–25.

17 Gorst-Unsworth C, Goldenberg E. Psychological sequelae of torture and organised violence by refugees from Iraq. *Br J Psychiatry.* 1998; **172**: 90–94.

18 Steel Z, Silove D, Phan T *et al.* Long-term effect of psychological trauma on the mental health of refugees resettled in Australia: a population-based study. *Lancet.* 2002; **360**: 1056–62.

19 Mollica RF, Caspi-Yavin Y, Bollini P *et al.* The Harvard Trauma Questionnaire: validating a cross-cultural instrument for measuring torture, trauma, and post-traumatic stress disorder in Indochinese refugees. *J Nerv Ment Dis.* 1992; **180**: 111–16.

20 Sinnerbrink I, Silove DM, Manicavasagar VL *et al.* Asylum seekers: general health status and problems with access to health care. *Med J Aust.* 1996; **165**: 634–7.

21 Silove D, Sinnerbrink I, Field A *et al*. Anxiety, depression and PTSD in asylum-seekers: association with pre-migration trauma and post-migration stressors. *Br J Psychiatry*. 1997; **170**: 351–7.

22 Turner SW, Bowie C, Dunn G *et al*. Mental health of Kosovan refugees in the UK. *Br J Psychiatry*. 2003; **182**: 444–8.

23 Carlson E, Rosser-Hogan R. Trauma experiences, post-traumatic stress, dissociation and depression in Cambodian refugees. *Am J Psychiatry*. 1991; **148**: 1548–51.

24 Weine SM, Becker DF, McGlashan TH *et al*. Psychiatric consequences of 'ethnic cleansing': clinical assessments and trauma testimonies of newly resettled Bosnian refugees. *Am J Psychiatry*. 1995; **152**: 536–42.

25 Ai AL, Peterson C, Ubelhor D. War-related trauma and symptoms of post-traumatic stress disorder among adult Kosovar refugees. *J Trauma Stress*. 2002; **15**: 157–60.

26 Mollica RF, Wyshak G, Lavelle J. The psychosocial impact of war trauma on Southeast Asian refugees. *Am J Psychiatry*. 1987; **144**: 1567–72.

27 Hinton WL, Chen YC, Du N *et al*. DSM–III disorders in Vietnamese refugees. Prevalence and correlates. *J Nerv Ment Dis*. 1991; **181**: 113–22.

28 Hondius AJK, van Willigen LHM, Kleijn WC *et al*. Health problems among Latin-American and Middle-Eastern Refugees in the Netherlands: relations with violence exposure and ongoing socio-psychological strain. *J Trauma Stress*. 2000; **13**: 619–34.

29 Blair R. Risk factors associated with PTSD and major depression among Cambodian refugees in Utah. *Health Soc Work*. 2000; **25**: 23–30.

30 Ferrada-Noli M, Asberg M, Ormstad K *et al*. Suicidal behavior after severe trauma. Part 1. PTSD diagnoses, psychiatric comorbidity and assessments of suicidal behavior. *J Trauma Stress*. 1998; **11**: 103–12.

31 Clarke G, Sack WH, Goff B. Three forms of stress in Cambodian adolescent refugees. *J Abnorm Child Psychol*. 1993; **21**: 65–77.

32 De Vries J. *Psychosociale Hulpverlening en Vluchtelingen [Psychosocial Assistance and Refugees]*. Utrecht: Stichting Pharos; 2000.

33 Cragg RD. *Drugs Scoping Study. Asylum seekers and refugee communities*. London: Home Office; 2003.

34 Wildschut J, Lempens A, van der Most D *et al*. *Asielzoekers, Vluchtelingen en Illegalen in de Utrechtse Harddrugscene. Een onderzoek naar de omvang, kenmerken en positie van niet-westerse harddruggebruikers die afkomstig zijn uit andere dan de Nederlandse immigratielanden [Asylum Seekers, Refugees and People Without Papers in the Hard Drug Scene of Utrecht, The Netherlands. A study on the extent, characteristics and position of non-Western hard drug users originating from countries other than the Dutch immigration countries]*. Rotterdam: Instituut voor Verslavingsonderzoek (Institute for Addiction Research); 2003.

35 Williams CL, Berry JW. Primary prevention of acculturative stress among refugees. *Am Psychol*. 1991; **46**: 632–41.

36 Kivling-Bodén G, Sundbom E. The relationship between post-traumatic stress symptoms and life in exile in a clinical group of refugees from the former Yugoslavia. *Acta Psychiatr Scand*. 2002; **105**: 461–8.

37 Hauf E, Vaglum P. Organised violence and the stress of exile as predictors of mental health in a community cohort of Vietnamese refugees three years after resettlement. *Br J Psychiatry*. 1995; **166**: 360–7.

38 Momartin S, Silove D, Manicavasagar V *et al*. Dimensions of trauma associated with post-traumatic stress disorder (PTSD) caseness, severity and functional impairment: a study of Bosnian refugees resettled in Australia. *Soc Sci Med*. 2003; **57**: 775–81.

39 Whittington D, Abdi S. Somali substance misuse: causes and impacts; www.orexis.org.uk/Research.htm (accessed 1 April 2006).

40 Miller KE, Worthington GJ, Muzurovic J *et al*. Bosnian refugees and the stressors of exile: a narrative study. *Am J Orthopsychiatry*. 2002; **72**: 341–54.

41 Terheggen MA, Stroebe MS, Kleber RJ. Western conceptualisations and eastern experience: a cross-cultural study of traumatic stress reactions among Tibetan refugees in India. *J Trauma Stress*. 2001; **14**: 391–403.

42 Sundquist K, Johansson LM, DeMarinis V *et al*. Post-traumatic stress disorder and psychiatric comorbidity: symptoms in a random sample of female Bosnian refugees. *Eur Psychiatry*. 2005; **20**: 158–64.

43 Thulesius H, Håkansson A. Screening for post-traumatic stress disorder symptoms among Bosnian refugees. *J Trauma Stress*. 1999; **12**: 167–74.

44 Beiser M, Hou F. Language acquisition, unemployment and depressive disorder among Southeast Asian refugees: a 10-year study. *Soc Sci Med*. 2001; **53**: 1321–34.

45 Pernice R, Brook J. Refugees' and immigrants' mental health: association of demographic and post-immigration factors. *J Soc Psychol*. 1996; **136**: 511–19.

46 Beiser M, Johnson PJ, Turner RJ. Unemployment, underemployment and depressive affect among Southeast Asian refugees. *Psychol Med*. 1993; **23**: 731–43.

47 Sourander A. Refugee families during asylum seeking. *Nord J Psychiatry*. 2003; **57**: 203–7.

48 Nabuzoka D, Badhadhe FA. Use and perceptions of khat among young Somalis in a UK city. *Addiction Res*. 2000; **8**: 5–26.

49 Dupont HJ, Kaplan CD, Verbraeck HT *et al*. Killing time: drug and alcohol problems among asylum seekers in the Netherlands. *Int J Drug Policy*. 2005; **16**: 27–36.

50 Beiser M, Noh S, Feng H *et al*. Southeast Asian refugees' perceptions of racial discrimination in Canada. *Can Ethnic Stud*. 2001; **33**: 46–71.

51 Fountain J, editor. *Young Refugees and Asylum Seekers in Greater London: vulnerability to problematic drug use*. London: Greater London Authority; 2004.

52 Yee BWK, Thu ND. Correlates of drug use and abuse among Indochinese refugees: mental health correlates. *J Psychoactive Drugs*. 1987; **19**: 77–83.

53 Braam R, Dupont H, Verbraeck H. *Asielzoekers en Middelengebruik [Asylum Seekers and Substance Use]*. Utrecht: Centrum voor Verslavingsonderzoek; 1999.

54 D'Avanzo C, Frye B, Froman R. Culture, stress and substance use in Cambodian refugee women. *J Stud Alcohol*. 1994; **55**: 420–26.

55 Landschaftsverband Westfalen-Lippe (LWL). *SEARCH II. Materials for drug prevention for asylum seekers, refugees and illegal immigrants*; www.lwl.org/ks-download/downloads/searchII/SEARCH_II_e.pdf (accessed 13 April 2006).

56 Landschaftsverband Westfalen-Lippe (LWL). *SEARCH. Drug prevention for asylum seekers, refugees and illegal immigrants*; www.lwl.org/LWL/Jugend/KS/Publikationen/projekte/Search_Downloads/search_downloads_english (accessed 13 April 2006).

Chapter 7

A cultural approach to understanding the stigma of drug use: the experience of prisoners in England and Wales

Sundari Anitha

Sociologists and criminologists have utilised the concepts of labelling, deviance and stigma in their investigations into the influence of social structure on individual action and identity.[1,2] For example, in his influential work, Howard Becker argues that the label 'deviant' is based on the reactions and responses of others to what is viewed as a fundamental flaw on the part of an individual.[3] Later sociologists have criticised the assumption of a monolithic consensus to which an individual fails to conform, thereby acquiring the label of a deviant. They have argued that social values themselves are pluralistic, and that labelling is one of the ways in which those who hold dominant positions within the structures of power recast the social world. Jock Young, for instance, examines the role of the media in constructing social policies, meanings and moral panic related to drug use, thereby amplifying the deviance.[4]

The concept of stigma has also been examined in relation to mental health, other illness, drug use and problematic drug use,[a] where the focus has largely been on the manifestations and medical and psychosocial consequence of stigma, both for individuals and for the provision of services. Drugs researchers and drug service providers have in particular used this concept to understand attitudes to drug use among Black and minority ethnic populations,[5,b] as well as the barriers to accessing services, but have paid little attention to the meanings and dimensions of stigma. This chapter will look at manifestations of stigma related to problematic drug use in prisons in an attempt to understand how the experience of stigma is mediated by social circumstances and cultural context.

Stigma refers to a negative attribute, trait or disorder that marks out or labels its bearer as different from 'normal' people and that attracts social sanctions.[1,6] The construction of stereotypes about the 'other' makes it easier for 'normal' people to distance themselves from and discriminate against the stigmatised.[7] The media plays a crucial role in the construction and reinforcement of these stereotypes.[8–10] Over the centuries, and across different cultures, the markers that attract social sanction have ranged from leprosy to mental illness,[11] but the attribution of a link between the stigmatising marker and the moral worth of the individual, and often, by extension, to those associating with the stigmatised, has not changed.

The term 'stigma' captures a combination of feelings, such as shame, blame, secrecy and low self-esteem, which are perceived by the stigmatised and their associates and indicate society's judgement and exclusion of them.[12,13] As in the case of mental illness, the stigma attached to the problematic use of drugs appears to prevent some people who need help from seeking it, due to internalised feelings of shame or fear of rejection by society,[14–16] and it also hinders many who do seek help from deriving lasting benefit from their treatment.[17]

Methods

This chapter draws upon the research conducted by the Centre for Ethnicity and Health on the delivery of prison drug services in England and Wales, with a focus on Black and minority ethnic prisoners.[18] The aims of the study were to identify the factors that facilitate or hinder access to prison drug services, to distinguish those factors that affect Black and minority ethnic prisoners, and to provide recommendations for areas of work that require attention.

In order to achieve the study's aims, the project reviewed relevant literature in order to identify themes for the research instruments, collated the available relevant statistical data, mapped the existing prison drug services, and explored a range of perspectives on the issues surrounding this provision. Data were collected from a total of 334 individuals, who were interviewed, completed questionnaires or participated in focus groups. They included interviews in eight prisons with 149 prisoners (51% of whom were from Black and minority ethnic communities), prison officers, prison drug workers, members of prison Independent Monitoring Boards, prison drug service planners, commissioners and providers, ex-prisoners from Black and minority ethnic communities, members of Black and minority ethnic communities, and representatives of organisations working with prisoners, ex-prisoners and their families.

Implications of stigma for prisoners, their families and their communities

The possible explanations for the stigma attached to mental illness have been identified as the perceived dangerousness of the patient, the attribution of responsibility for their illness to the patient, poor prognosis and disruption of social interaction with 'normal' people.[19] Similarly, studies on the attitudes towards HIV status and AIDS reveal that they mirror the stigma attached to problematic drug use, because the stigma in these cases is often associated with the perceived mode of transmission – via either sexual activity or intravenous drug users sharing injecting equipment – and the perception that the illness is a consequence of deviant behaviour, symptomatic of moral defects.[20,21] For instance, Crandall notes the particular stigmatisation of HIV status and AIDS in an intravenous drug user compared with a blood-transfusion recipient or a healthcare worker who contracted the disease accidentally.[22] Fife and Wright have made similar observations with regard to the stigma associated with cancer and HIV and AIDS.[23] These observations about attitudes to mental illness and HIV and AIDS can be transferred to problematic drug use, which is particularly likely to be viewed by society as self-inflicted.[24]

However, do all societies view the problematic use of drugs as self-inflicted? In the context of mental illness, it has been suggested that the value placed on the autonomous individual in industrialised, largely western cultures attributes individual personal culpability for the illness, which therefore shapes the social response to it in the form of stigmatisation of the individual.[25] Although the family, associates and community of white drug users may indeed stigmatise them on account of their drug use, this stigma, even if it is understood in the context of their family background or a deprivation narrative of the community, is attached to the autonomous individual, as is the ultimate responsibility for his or her behaviour. Is there an additional dimension to the stigma experienced by drug users from Black and minority ethnic populations?

In communities from South Asia (India, Pakistan, Bangladesh and Sri Lanka), for example, the individual is not necessarily viewed as autonomous but is defined, at least in part, by their role and position within a wider network of kinship ties and family relationships, and by their ability to function within the parameters of those roles. The corollary of this is that these significant others are also responsible for maintaining this close network of relationships and the rules governing morality within this context. Any failing is that of this collective, rather than just that of the individual. Given this, the attribution of stigma attached to the use of drugs, rather than being ascribed to the autonomous individual, may be felt among the family, a wider network of associates or indeed the whole community, which would experience the loss of status or the social sanctions that stigma attracts as shame and dishonour.[26,27] This is more than an exaggerated version of the stigma by association with the stigmatised person that is referred to by Goffman,[1] because the stigma here cannot be shaken off by ending that association. It is qualitatively different because it attaches to an entity that is larger than an individual.

The research in prisons discussed here revealed that for some male Black and minority ethnic prisoners, fear of the family or the community discovering their drug use was an important factor in preventing them from accessing drug services. The study participants also highlighted the cultural and religious attitudes towards ex-prisoners, particularly if they were also drug users, that prevented them from re-establishing relationships with family, friends and the wider community. Although it is not clear whether these are issues that affect solely Black and minority ethnic prisoners, the issue was raised most often by individuals from South Asian communities. Focus groups with members of Black and minority ethnic communities and interviews with representatives of organisations working with prisoners, ex-prisoners and their families revealed that such concerns were not unfounded:

> It's very difficult [for an ex-prisoner] to get back into society. Getting a job and acceptance in the community is really difficult. Even access to the mosque . . . If someone wants to change, society doesn't let them.
>
> (Community member, Indian)

> I have not approached drug services, in or out [of prison], because I did not want anyone to know I was a junkie. If I went to a clinic or a rehab, everyone would know and it would bring disrespect to my family and to me. That is why my parents still don't know about my drug use.
>
> (Male prisoner, Pakistani)

The experience of stigma in a prison culture

As discussed above, stigma marks out its bearer as different from 'normal.' However, what constitutes normal behaviour varies according to the society in which it occurs. Therefore, just as behaviour that is stigmatised by some ethnic groups may be seen as normal by others, the stigma attached to certain behaviour outside prisons may be exaggerated inside them. Prison represents a unique society in which the prisoners are subject to an official discourse of control and order through the exercise of discipline, the precise regulation of day-to-day activities and the identification of non-compliant individuals as 'problem prisoners.'[28] In this context, there is very little that prisoners can do to alter the 'grant of power without equal'[29] that prison administrators hold, or to shift the balance of power between themselves and prison officers.[30] Thus the importance of status among peers, which can be controlled to some extent, becomes very exaggerated.

Swann and James[31] have noted how stigma can lead to under-reporting of drug problems by prisoners, as the fear of rejection by their peers and their application of social sanctions may act as barriers to accessing drug services. In the study reported here, this was an issue that was seen to particularly affect male prisoners, especially young males, for whom 'appearances in the very masculine environment of prison are vital'[32] and approaching services could be interpreted by others as a sign of weakness:

> Some people don't like seeing the prison drugs service or talking to them, or others knowing you have a problem . . . are trying to get help.
>
> (Prison officer)

> Lots of people here need drug services, but few ask. This is because of the stigma of being seen to ask for help. This is seen as being weak – it is a macho thing. Everyone wants to be seen as a big hard man.
>
> (Prisoner, white British)

Stigma is not a uniform concept, nor is it experienced in a one-dimensional way. The experience of stigma by an individual, family or community is subjective and is mediated by the cultural context, the nature of the stigmatising factor and the social circumstances. In the context of a male prison, any attempt to shed the stigmatising factor by accessing drug treatment services may also be fraught with the danger of losing social status, as seeking help in this way could be seen as flouting the dominant discourse of masculinity and invulnerability.

The multidimensionality of stigma

Early studies on stigma focused on it as a negative attribute that afflicts the passive victim.[13] Recent studies have shifted the focus to society rather than the attributes of the individual per se,[6,33] and in recognition of the social dynamic and power structures at play, have explored the perspectives, coping mechanisms and experiences of the stigmatised, viewing them as constructors of their own reality.[34,35] The attribution of stigma seeks to impose a power deficit on the recipient by conferring an inferior status through social sanction or isolation. However, as Certeau argues, structures of power seldom invoke unmediated acceptance from those disadvantaged by the power imbalance.[36] In the day-to-day arena of power relationships, the actors actively assume ambivalent and multiple positions – from acquiescence to rejection, from negotiation to replication – as they seek to construct a buffering life space, and Crocker et al.[37] have examined how individuals do this as they seek to protect themselves from the effects of stigma by attributing it to prejudice.

In the prisons that were visited for the study reported here, some male prisoners responded to multiple dimensions of the stigma of drug use, as well as to the stigma of help seeking for problematic drug use, often from women service providers, by claiming that they managed their drug use without service interventions, or that they were strong enough to do so should they wish. There were others who showed a preference for engaging with peer support groups, thus negotiating a space for disclosure where they would be among equals. Yet others made a mitigating case by attributing greater stigma to users of drugs other than those that they were using themselves.

Prisoners, prison officers and drug workers reported that allied to concerns about confidentiality, attitudes to the use of certain drugs prevented prisoners, especially Black and minority ethnic prisoners, from accessing drug services. Many Black and minority ethnic prisoners were concerned that if they approached the prison drug services, other prisoners would discover their drug use and bully or ostracise them. The study found that the level of concern about stigma was linked to the choice of drug. Younger prisoners were more likely than older ones to report stigma attached to the use of drugs, apart from cannabis – there was little evidence of stigma attached to cannabis use in any age group. The use of heroin and crack cocaine attracted particular stigma among many prisoners of all ages, but such views were expressed most strongly and most often by Black and minority ethnic inmates. Due to fear of social sanctions, bullying and/or internalisation of feelings of shame, black and minority ethnic prisoners were generally prepared to disclose crack cocaine use in order to access services, but were less keen to disclose heroin use, especially if they injected the drug:

> They [prisoners] are ashamed to let others know they use [heroin] because they would diss [disrespect] you.
>
> (Prisoner, black British)

> Many of the black lads may not want to admit to using heroin – even crack use is a problem, but admitting to heroin use will be a complete loss of face. There is a lot of posturing here – they don't want to be seen as weak in front of each other.
>
> (Prison drug worker)

> I use heroin but do not think that other black people should inject heroin. If others here knew you were injecting, you would get no ratings, no respect. It's bad enough taking heroin, but injecting . . .
>
> (Prisoner, black British)

It could be argued when users of crack cocaine cite the greater stigma accruing to users of heroin, who in turn point to injectors of heroin, that apart from being a continuum of social attitudes outside prison,[38] prisoners are trying to deflect some of the stigma from themselves to others whose identities are even more spoiled than theirs, and at the same time replicating the stigmatisation that they themselves often receive. Similarly, a response that was encountered among Black and minority ethnic prisoners with regard to cannabis use was that it is comparable to alcohol use among white communities, or indeed that alcohol is the more dangerous drug and should attract social sanction.

Understanding stigma: the case for culturally competent service providers

For some Black and minority ethnic prisoners, the predominantly white composition of prison drug service teams is another barrier to accessing their services. Gooden suggests that 'pride is often the last thing given up by African-Caribbean and Asian cultures',[39] and the findings of the present study support this:

> Lots of black users don't ask for help because they are ashamed to admit they have a problem. If black staff were delivering services, they might be able to talk to them.
>
> (Prisoner, black Caribbean)

> It [not accessing services] is mostly about the authorities knowing. They cannot relate to the white authority figures . . . they cannot relate to those delivering the services – seen as all-white authority figures.
>
> (Prisoner, Pathan)

The experience of stigma and the prisoners' responses to it here seem to be complex and often contradictory. Many Black and minority ethnic prisoners reported fear of being stigmatised by their peers, family and community, and this feeling often extends to drug workers from their community, who they may be reluctant to approach. At the same time, predominantly white drug service teams are also a barrier to access for these prisoners. What they seem to be arguing for are visible signs of the cultural competence of the drug service providers,[40,41] either through the presence of an ethnically diverse staff team or through visible, proactive measures to make the service accessible. Perceptions of procedural justice, consistent outcomes, and regular, efficient service delivery greatly increase the likelihood of the prisoners granting legitimacy to the service. Scraton et al.[42] argue that prisons, with their unrelenting imposition of authority, must inevitably lack legitimacy, and others have argued that a conflict between custody and therapy is also inevitable.[43,44] However, whereas incarceration itself relies on 'the full potential of state coercion',[42] as far as day-to-day regimes, routines and services are concerned, only legitimate social arrangements generate normative commitments towards compliance and engagement.[45-47]

Following on from Sparks and Bottom's analysis of the problem of legitimacy in prison,[41] it could be argued from the findings of the study that every time a prison officer shouts out publicly to a prisoner 'drug service to see you', thus exposing their drug use and help seeking, every time prisoners perceive that they could not approach drug services at a group induction because of the stigma associated with help seeking, and did not get the chance to access services later in their sentence, and every time the only aftercare referral that is possible is in the home community of a prisoner fearful of community sanctions because of drug use, an inherent legitimacy crisis is created. Despite the difficulties of achieving complete confidentiality in the context of a prison, and the resource implications of individual induction sessions, culturally competent drug service providers who can understand concerns about stigma and take proactive measures to improve drug service accessibility would go a long way towards addressing some prisoners' concerns.

Conclusion

The findings reported above are also applicable to other Black and minority ethnic communities in Europe. In a study that examined drug use among these populations, the failure of drug users and their families to admit to a drug problem because of the associated shame was noted among the Roma/Sinti in Austria and Germany, Moroccans and especially Turkish people in the Netherlands, Black and minority ethnic groups in Norway, gypsies in Portugal and (especially when the drug user was female) in Spain, Iranian males in Sweden, several Black and minority ethnic groups in the UK.[48] Another example of different cultural sensitivities in that study was that Black and minority ethnic communities in Sweden reported stigma attached to seeking any help from social services, especially for drug use. Although targeting drug services at the needs of diverse communities would help to overcome some of the barriers to accessing these services, in some countries this is either constitutionally forbidden (e.g. in France and Portugal) or the issue of cultural diversity does not appear to be addressed in relation to drug services (e.g. in Germany, the Netherlands, Spain and Sweden).[48]

I shall end with an example that indicates how a consideration of the effects and fear of stigma can make a difference to the planning and delivery of prison drug services. During my discussions with a prison Area Drug Coordinator (ADC, responsible for drug policy implementation at regional level), she referred to what she had initially perceived as a successful venture in the prisons in her area. The prison drug services operated a stall in the visitors' room in order to engage the family in the treatment of drug-using prisoners, hoping that this would be an added source of support for the prisoners. However, after seeing the report on the study discussed in this chapter, the ADC wondered what impact this might be having on South Asian prisoners. If a prisoner has kept their drug use secret from their family because of fear of the stigma it would incur, would a public greeting from a drug service provider jeopardise their relationship with their family? If there was more than one South Asian family visiting the prison, would gossip that a family had been talking to a drug service provider affect their status within the community? And were fears of such breaches of confidentiality preventing other South Asian prisoners from accessing prison drug services?

Stigma is experienced in many different ways by drug users, and being aware of these multiple strands would enable prison drug service providers to address the issue as a barrier to accessing services. Such awareness would enable them to provide a culturally competent service that meets the needs of drug users from ethnically diverse communities.

Endnotes

a In this chapter, problematic drug use refers to 'the illegal or illicit drug taking . . . which leads a person to experience social, psychological, physical or legal problems related to intoxication or regular excessive consumption and/or dependence . . . drug taking which causes harm to the individual, their significant others [such as their family or partner] or the wider community.'[49]

b Of the various terms that are used to refer to the many diverse communities in Europe, the author prefers the term 'Black and minority ethnic communities.' This reflects the position of the Centre for Ethnicity and Health, whose concern is not only with those for whom 'Black' is a political term, denoting those who identify around a basis of skin colour distinction or who may face discrimination because of this or their culture. 'Black and minority ethnic' also acknowledges the diversity that exists within these communities, and includes a wider range of those who may not consider their identity to be Black, but who nevertheless constitute a distinct ethnic group.

References

1 Goffman I. *Stigma: notes on the management of spoiled identity*. Harmondsworth: Penguin Books; 1990.
2 Matza D. *Becoming Deviant*. Englewood Cliffs, NJ: Prentice-Hall Mayer; 1969.
3 Becker H. *Outsiders: studies in the sociology of deviance*. New York: Free Press; 1963.
4 Young J. *The Drug Takers*. London: Paladin; 1971.
5 Fountain J, Bashford J, Underwood S *et al. Update and Complete Analysis of Drug Use, Consequences and Correlates Amongst Minorities. Volume 1. Synthesis.* Lisbon: European Monitoring Centre for Drugs and Drug Addiction; 2002.

6 Ainlay S, Becker G, Coleman L. *The Dilemma of Difference: a multidisciplinary view of stigma*. New York: Plenum Press; 1986.

7 Byrne P. The stigma of mental illness and ways of diminishing it. *Adv Psychiatr Treat*. 2000; **6**: 65–72.

8 Cape GS. Addiction, stigma and movies. *Acta Psychiatr Scand*. 2003; **107**: 163–9.

9 Wilson C, Nairn R, Coverdale J, Franzcp *et al.* How mental illness is portrayed in children's television: a prospective study. *Br J Psychiatry*. 2000; **176**: 440–3.

10 Radford T. Influence and power of the media. *Lancet*. 1996; **347**: 1533–5.

11 Porter R. Can the stigma of mental illness be changed? *Lancet*. 1998; **352**: 1049–50.

12 Kurzban R, Leary MR. Evolutionary origins of stigmatisation: the functions of social exclusion. *Psychol Bull*. 2001; **127**: 187–208.

13 Cumming J, Cumming E. On the stigma of mental illness. *Commun Ment Health J*. 1965; **1**: 135–43.

14 Lowe A. The stigma attached to substance misuse. *Practice Nurse*. 2000; **19**: 436–41.

15 Royal College of Psychiatrists, Royal College of Physicians of London and British Medical Association. *Mental Illness: stigmatisation and discrimination within the medical profession. Council Report CR91*. Glasgow: Bell and Bail Ltd; 2001.

16 Social Exclusion Unit. *Report. Mental health and social exclusion*. London: Office of the Deputy Prime Minister; 2004.

17 Link BG, Struening EL, Rahav M *et al.* On stigma and its consequences: evidence from a longitudinal study of men with dual diagnoses of mental illness and substance abuse. *J Health Soc Behav*. 1997; **38**: 177–90.

18 Fountain J, Roy A, Anitha S *et al. Issues Surrounding the Delivery of Drug Services in England and Wales, with a Focus on Black and Minority Ethnic Prisoners*. London: Prison Service Drug Strategy Unit/Home Office; 2004.

19 Hayward P, Bright JA. Stigma of mental illness: review and critique. *J Ment Health*. 1997; **6**: 345–54.

20 Lichtenstein B. Caught at the clinic: African-American men, stigma and STI treatment in the Deep South. *Gender Society*. 2004; **18**: 369–88.

21 Taylor B. HIV, stigma and health: integration of theoretical concepts and the live experiences of individuals. *J Adv Nurs*. 2001; **35**: 792–8.

22 Crandall CS. Multiple stigma and AIDS: illness, stigma and attitudes toward homosexuals and IV drug users in AIDS-related stigmatization. *J Commun Appl Soc Psychiatry*. 1991; **1**: 165–75.

23 Fife BL, Wright ER. The dimensionality of stigma: a comparison of its impact on the self of persons with HIV/AIDS and cancer. *J Health Soc Behav*. 2000; **41**: 50–67.

24 Crisp AH, Geelder MG, Rix S *et al.* Stigmatisation of people with mental illnesses. *Br J Psychiatry*. 2000; **177**: 4–7.

25 Littlewood R. Cultural variation in the stigmatisation of mental illness. *Lancet*. 1998; **352**: 1056–7.

26 Wanigaratne S, Dar K, Abdulrahim D *et al.* Ethnicity and drug use: exploring the nature of particular relationships among diverse populations in the United Kingdom. *Drugs Educ Prev Policy*. 2003; **10**: 39–55.

27 Weiss SRB, Kung H-C, Pearson J. Emerging issues in gender and ethnic differences in substance abuse and treatment. *Curr Women's Health Rep*. 2003; **3**: 245–53.

28 King RS, McDermott K. 'My geranium is subversive': some notes on the management of trouble in prisons. *Br J Sociol*. 1990; **41**: 445–71.

29 Sykes G. *The Society of Captives*. Princeton, NJ: Princeton University Press; 1958.

30 Sparks JR, Bottoms AE. Legitimacy and order in prisons. *Br J Sociol*. 1995; **46**: 45–62.

31 Swann R, James P. The effect of the prison environment on inmate drug-taking behaviour. *Howard J*. 1998; **37**: 252–65.

32 Cope N. Drug use in prison: the experience of young offenders. *Drugs Educ Prev Policy*. 2000; **7**: 355–66.

33 Sayce L. Stigma, discrimination and social exclusion: what's in a word? *J Ment Health*. 1998; **7**: 331–43.

34 Miller CT, Kaiser CR. A theoretical perspective on coping with stigma. *J Soc Issues*. 2001; **57**: 73–92.

35 Oyserman D, Swim JK. Stigma: an insider's view. *J Soc Issues*. 2001; **57**: 1–14.

36 Certeau MD. *The Practice of Everyday Life* (translated by Rendall S). Berkeley, CA: University of California Press; 1984.

37 Crocker J, Kristin V, Maria T *et al*. Social stigma: the affective consequences of attributional ambiguity. *J Pers Soc Psychol*. 1991; **60**: 218–28.

38 Borrill J, Maden A, Martin A *et al*. *The Differential Substance Misuse Treatment Needs of Women, Ethnic Minorities and Young Offenders in Prison: prevalence of substance misuse and treatment needs*. Home Office Online Report 33/03. London: Home Office; 2003.

39 Gooden T. *Carers and Parents of African-Caribbean and Asian Substance Users in Nottingham: a needs analysis. Final report*. Nottingham: Organisational Change Innovation Development (ORCHID)/Nottingham Black Initiative (NBI); 1999.

40 Fountain J, Bashford J, Winters M *et al*. *Black and Minority Ethnic Communities in England: a review of the literature on drug use and related service provision*. London: National Treatment Agency; 2003.

41 Luger LD, Sookhoo D. Rapid needs assessment of the provision of drug and alcohol services for people from minority ethnic groups with drug and alcohol problems. *Diversity Health Soc Care*. 2005; **2**: 167–76.

42 Scraton P, Sim J, Skidmore P. *Prisons under Protest*. Buckingham: Open University Press; 1991.

43 Cloward RA, Cressey DR, Grosser GH *et al*. *Theoretical Studies in Social Organization of Prison*. New York: Social Science Research Council; 1960.

44 Swann R, James P. The effect of the prison environment on inmate drug-taking behaviour. *Howard J*. 1998; **37**: 252–65.

45 Sparks JR, Bottom AE. Legitimacy and order in prisons. *Br J Sociol*. 1995; **46**: 45–62.

46 Beetham D. *The Legitimation of Power*. London: Macmillan; 1991.

47 Tyler TR. *Why People Obey the Law*. New Haven, CT: Yale University Press; 1990.

48 Fountain J, Bashford J, Underwood S *et al*. *Update and Completion of the Analysis of Drug Use, Consequences and Correlates Amongst Minorities*. Lisbon: European Monitoring Centre for Drugs and Drug Addiction; 2002.

49 National Treatment Agency for Substance Misuse (NTA). *Models of Care for the Treatment of Drug Misusers. Part 2. Full reference report*; www.nta.nha.uk (accessed 20 May 2006).

Chapter 8

Diversification endangered

Alfred Springer

This chapter discusses how, in Austria, a special system of diversified maintenance treatment for opioid addicts has developed, allowing the prescription of different substances for maintenance purposes. This system seemed to work well and was accepted by the majority of medical doctors involved in this type of treatment, and also by their clients. The major drug prescribed has changed over the years, from methadone to slow-release morphine, since the majority of clients preferred the latter medication. However, in 2004 a campaign took place aimed at the abolition of the use of slow-release morphine preparations for maintenance purposes. The campaign stimulated a stigmatisation process that eventually had an impact on the formulation of an amendment of the Austrian regulations concerning the implementation of maintenance treatment. The use of slow-release formulated morphine will possibly be prohibited, putting an end to the Austrian method of diversified medical treatment of opioid dependency.

Methods

This chapter is based partly on participant observation and partly on the systematic analysis of documents from diverse sources, including the campaign against the use of slow-release morphine for maintenance purposes, media reports on drug fatalities and on maintenance treatment, press releases, press conferences, and the draft of an amendment to Austrian drug laws (the Substitution Act). The media analysis covers the period from April 2004 to December 2005, when the print media wrote extensively about drug-related issues, focusing on deaths, and daily newspapers from all Austrian regions were collected and analysed. Labelling theory and the theory of stigmatisation are used as a reference frame for the interpretation of the process described and the conclusions drawn. Despite some criticism concerning its relevance,[1] the deviance model has long been used in sociological and criminological interpretations of illicit drug use and its implications,[2] and remains a widely accepted approach to explaining the phenomenon.

The deviance model is also very useful for understanding the societal processes triggered by maintenance treatment, and in 1974 Miller extended the conceptualisation and definition of primary and secondary deviance to describe the social status of the maintenance client.[3] He created a third category of deviance, 'tertiary deviance', to explain the stigma associated with methadone maintenance in relation to heroin addiction, which can be defined as secondary deviance since it develops within a deviancy amplification spiral. Furthermore, many aspects of the lifestyle of addicted individuals and the life cycle of addiction can be interpreted as an adaptation to the societal response to the primary deviance of drug taking. Miller defined tertiary deviance as the societal solution to social problems that takes the form of concentrating upon eliminating or minimising the negative effects of secondary deviance, as opposed to previous efforts to eliminate primary deviance. According to Miller's interpretation, the tertiary deviance solution leads to a kind of 'semi-deviance', with the clients being maintained on opioid substances. Later observations and descriptions by, for example, Kallen,[4] Acker,[5] Murphy and Irwin[6] and Joseph[7] were consistent with this.

The early concept of tertiary deviance was tailored to the interpretation of the fate of drug users. It differs somewhat from Kitsuse's later, more widely used concept of tertiary deviance.[8] Kitsuse suggested the term 'tertiary deviant' (in contrast to primary and secondary deviant) to describe someone who presses for re-definition of deviant conduct in order to change standards for acceptable behaviour and/or who searches for support to defend a deviant identity. The concepts of Miller and Kitsuse are therefore dissimilar. In Kitsuse's model the term 'tertiary deviance' signifies an action (the activities of the stigmatised groups or individuals), whereas in Miller's model it describes a societal reaction and a rather passive state of the stigmatised group or individual, resulting from ongoing stigmatisation. The relabelling issue, crucial to Kitsuse's approach, is absent from Miller's conceptualisation. Clinard and Meiers are among those who adopted Kitsuse's definition – that tertiary deviance is an attempt to relabel deviant behaviour as non-deviant.[9]

Maintenance treatment: state and status

Since its introduction during the 1980s, maintenance treatment of opiate addiction has become a major element in the medical treatment of drug abuse across Europe. For example, in 2003, more than half a million substance abusers in the European Union (EU) were undergoing this treatment.[10] After some initial resistance, maintenance treatment has come to be regarded as an effective way to reduce the problems associated with heroin addiction. This view is clearly expressed in official documents by the European Monitoring Centre for Drugs and Drug Addiction (EMCDDA),[10] the Council of Europe's Pompidou Group,[11] the European Commission[12] and the World Health Organization.[13,14] Most evaluations have shown that, when correctly implemented, the treatment is capable of producing remarkable improvements in clients who were previously dysfunctional heroin addicts. Maintenance clients throughout the world have been restored to productive lives, their relationships with their families and children have been re-established, and many have resumed their education, obtained employment, and experienced an improvement in their physical and mental health.[7,12,15,16]

On the other hand, the criticism of this treatment concept, which began in its early days and was directed at Dole and Nyswander and their pioneering use of methadone, has not abated. Despite scientific evidence, maintenance treatment remains a controversial issue among substance abuse treatment providers, representatives of national, regional and local health authorities, policy makers, the public at large and the medical profession.[7] The criticism extends the prejudice associated with heroin addiction, and is the foundation for the stigma that is now attached to any type of maintenance treatment. Extensive clinic regulations enacted by state and local authorities to control maintenance treatment are, in essence, extensions of federal, state and local laws and drug policies to control heroin addicts and the process of addiction in the shadow of the 'War on Drugs.'

The stigma associated with maintenance treatment is derived from the transfer of deviance associated with heroin addiction,[3,5,7] inducing a state of tertiary deviance. In 1974, Miller had already identified the possible shortcomings of the 'tertiary deviance solution' as he understood it. He pointed out that methadone treatment should help to destigmatise the opioid-dependent individual, otherwise the stigma is transferred from the state of heroin addiction to the state of methadone maintenance. Miller concluded that this process indicates that the original ideological debate over the primary deviance has not been resolved, and his interpretation was supported by Murphy and Irwin in 1992.[6] In a review of three qualitative studies conducted in the 1980s, these authors described methadone clients as having a 'marginal identity', where they saw themselves – and were viewed by society – as deviant, despite their efforts to end their addiction. Like Miller, they found that the stigma attached to being in treatment for heroin addiction interferes with the process of normalisation that maintenance aims to achieve.

The concept of multidimensional diversification

When the concept of maintenance treatment was imported from the USA in the 1980s, prescription of methadone was the first (and sometimes the only) option available in Europe. Later, other types of opioid substitutes appeared on the European treatment scene. 'Diversification' became an influential slogan in the discourse on treatment approaches at both the professional and the political level. Currently, diversified prescription is considered to be a strategy for attracting clients and keeping them in treatment. This strategy seems to be essential for treatment-related aims as they are defined in the European Action Plan against Drugs.[17]

I have previously developed the concept of 'multidimensional diversification',[18] which allows the identification of different layers of diversification. According to this concept, diversification can take place with regard to the substance, the route of administration, and the size, scope and composition of maintenance programmes. Currently, across Europe, the substances prescribed include methadone, slow-release morphine/codeine, immediate-release morphine (heroin)/codeine, and buprenorphine, and their prescribed route of administration may be oral, nasal, by inhalation or by injection.

Diversified prescribing in Europe

The implementation of diversification mirrors the cultural ambivalence towards the medical interpretation of opioid dependency. Most often, diversification takes place only with regard to substances. An overview of the European region therefore shows a varied picture with regard to prescribed substances and routes of administration. In the various member states of the EU there is no consensus with regard to maintenance strategies.

According to the overview shown in Table 8.1, diversification of prescribed substances occurs in most European countries, whereas diversification of route of administration remains controversial. Usually the diverse substances are prescribed for oral use, and the prescription of injectable preparations is limited to experimental trials and/or is strictly controlled, requires special licensing and demands supervised consumption. Diversification with regard to route of administration has to be an issue of concern, because the route affects the bioavailability of a substance, and therefore its effects. The highest level of bioavailability is guaranteed by injection. Oral ingestion and 'chasing the dragon' (a form of inhalation) offer good bioavailability, whereas the smoking of cigarettes containing a substance produces only medium bioavailability.

Table 8.1: Diversified maintenance prescribing in some European countries

Oral methadone	Injectable methadone	Codeine/ dihydrocodeine	Slow-release morphine	Oral heroin	Injectable heroin	Buprenorphine	Other
Austria		Austria	Austria			Austria	
Belgium		Belgium					
Denmark						Denmark	
Finland						Finland	
France			France			France	
Germany		Germany			Germany	Germany	
Italy						Italy	
Luxembourg	Netherlands	Luxembourg					Luxembourg (Mephenon)
Netherlands					Netherlands	Netherlands	
Norway						Norway	
Portugal						Portugal	
Spain				Spain	Spain		
Sweden						Sweden	
Switzerland	Switzerland			Switzerland	Switzerland	Switzerland	
UK	UK			UK	UK		

Diversified prescribing in Austria

In Austria, 20,000 to 30,000 people are considered to be problematic drug consumers.[19] Medication-assisted treatment of opioid dependence with methadone was made available in 1987, followed by the official registration for that purpose of slow-release morphine and buprenorphine in 1998. A small proportion of substituted clients also receive codeine or dihydrocodeine in a slow-release formulation. The Austrian model is different from others in Europe because of the availability of different opioids for maintenance treatment. Until the latest developments, it also differed from other maintenance models with regard to the legal regulation of the dispersion of the substances. The Austrian Substitution Act makes them available under a common set of rules and regulations, and this derives from the interpretation of the nature of the drug problem. Since heroin addiction, like all other substance dependencies, is classified as an illness in Austria, substitution treatment represents a special form of an essentially medical intervention. According to this interpretation, diversified prescribing practices in Austria are following the rules of good medical practice. If a range of effective and suitable substances is available for the treatment of an illness, prescription cannot be restricted to one substance. It has to be matched with the characteristics and needs of the individual client.

During the course of the development of diversification, the prescription of methadone has been declining across Austria. Whereas in 2000, 53.4% of the total sample of maintenance clients received methadone, that proportion had decreased to 29.5% by 2002.[20] In 2004, 6,400 individuals were registered as receiving maintenance medications, of whom 2,890 (45.2%) were maintained on slow-release morphine preparations.[19,21] An analogous situation can be found in Vienna where, according to the Health Authority of Vienna, between November 2001 and May 2003 the rate of methadone prescriptions fell from 53% to 36%, while during the same period the rate of morphine prescriptions increased from 36% to 49%. Buprenorphine prescriptions in Vienna also increased from 10% in November 2001 to 14% in May 2003. During the same time period, maintenance treatment was increasingly administered by general practitioners (70% in 2001 and 76% in 2003), while the part played by specialised institutions decreased from 14% to 9%. Maintenance treatment by psychiatrists remained stable, in the range 15–16%. No special licensing is required for general practitioners who become involved in administering maintenance treatment, but continuing postgraduate training in issues related to the approach is necessary.

Research studies on the issues of quality of treatment and efficiency of diversification are scarce and not very well structured. The Ludwig–Boltzmann Institute for Addiction Research conducted a study on the early years of maintenance treatment in Austria,[22] there are reports about the Viennese drug scene in which users' assessments of diversified prescribing have been collected,[23,24] and a study comparing methadone and slow-release morphine in pregnancy.[25] Fischer *et al.*[26] and Kraigher *et al.*[27] conducted clinical studies in Vienna on the registration of slow-release morphine for maintenance purposes.

Although there have been unpublished conference presentations on diversified prescribing from treatment centres and on diversified maintenance in prison, there are no follow-up studies, no studies on the impact of maintenance, and none on those who drop out of treatment.

In most of the reports listed above, maintenance treatment with slow-release formulated morphine has been described and assessed as a viable, safe and efficient alternative to methadone. From interviews conducted within the Viennese drug scene, it was ascertained that individuals who were maintained on slow-release morphine preferred it to methadone, and their concomitant use of heroin appeared to be declining significantly. The prescription of slow-release morphine therefore seems to function as a kind of 'competitive prescribing', competing favourably with the substances on offer on the illegal market. The qualitative research conducted by the Viennese Social Projects supports this interpretation.[23,24]

Diversion of the prescribed substance has been identified as the major problem with regard to slow-release morphine maintenance prescription.[23,24] Some clients sell part of their daily dose in order to earn an income, often to buy other drugs, and oral preparations may be sold in order to buy injectable substances. Oral preparations may also be diverted by being injected, as oral maintenance cannot combat the craving for injecting that, in many cases, accompanies a dependency on opioids. The Austrian programme does not therefore represent an alternative to injecting maintenance programmes, and is not competing with programmes that prescribe diamorphine (heroin), including high dosages for intravenous use.

To a certain extent, the Austrian experience can be used as a model for the development of diversified oral opioid maintenance prescribing, avoiding the exorbitant costs both of control and of the experimental designs of heroin-prescribing trials. This conclusion has recently been confirmed in Australia.[28]

The campaign against slow-release morphine treatment

In 2004, a small group of concerned professionals, most of whom were involved in the treatment of substance-dependent individuals, challenged the use of slow-release morphine in maintenance treatment, and founded the *Interessensgemeinschaft Qualität in der Substitutions-behandlung* (Campaign for the Quality of Substitution Treatment). Their campaign was initiated by physicians, who were later joined by other medical professionals, social workers and a pharmacist. The campaigners were not completely opposed to the concept of mainte-nance, but they viewed it as a bridge to abstinence. Their concern had initially been stimulated by rumours that the intravenous use of pre-scribed oral preparations had led to an increase in the prevalence of open-heart surgery in the addicted population. Talcum as filling material in slow-release morphine was blamed for these alleged complications. However, this allegation was derived from the literature about such incidents in cases of intravenous use of amphetamines, especially of Ritalin (methylphenidate hydrochloride), in which the development of pulmonary arterial hypertension had been observed.

The campaign strategy

The group's campaign included attempts to:

- mobilise local agencies and professionals who had direct access to individuals within the target population
- bring together partnerships of public, voluntary and private sector bodies and professional organisations
- encourage local and national policy changes
- inform the public
- set an agenda for public debate about the topic in order to modify the climate of opinion about it
- involve the media as a communication tool.

The campaigners did not restrict their activities to Austria. They informed international bodies and experts, suggesting interventions at an international control level, and tried to recruit partners by sending their message to a broad range of institutions and individuals whom they considered to be potentially helpful for their aims. These included the United Nations control agencies, national and local health authorities and politicians, parents' organisations, and experts in medicine and social work from Austria and elsewhere. They found willing partners in some politicians, mostly on the right, and also used certain print media and local television to spread their message.

Features of the campaign

Awareness-raising campaigns are often based on fear-mongering issues. In this campaign, these could easily be identified. The prescription of morphine leads to addiction, an increase in the number of fatalities, the diversion of morphine, and adverse health consequences of intravenous administration, and it also serves as a gateway to addictive behaviour. Accusations brought forward to indict the use of slow-release morphine targeted the addict population as well as treatment providers and the pharmaceutical industry. It was implied by the campaign that prescribed morphine preparations for oral use were intravenously abused by a substantial proportion of the maintained population (the proportion quoted ranging from 20% to over 90%). With regard to diversion, it was suggested that, according to observations in many areas of Austria, slow-release morphine represented the 'Number One substance' on the illicit market. It was also proposed that diverted slow-release morphine preparations act as a gateway to problematic drug consumption for newcomers to the drug scene. Other accusations were made with regard to the morbidity and mortality of the addict population. Concern about the health consequences of intravenous abuse of slow-release morphine focused on cardiac complications and other – possibly deadly – consequences due to the ingredients of the oral medication blocking small vessels in the liver, kidney, lungs, heart valves and eyes of the clients. Last but not least, allegations were published which stated that up to 90% of fatal cases on the drug scene could be attributed to the abuse of slow-release morphine. In November 2004, Dr Gross, a general practitioner with a very large clientele of drug-addicted patients, prepared a leaflet in which she formulated 17 arguments to justify the immediate prohibition of slow-release morphine in maintenance treatment, and included all the above fear-mongering issues.

The campaign was remarkable in that it was not overtly directed against maintenance treatment as such (and as noted above, some of the key players were involved in providing this treatment). Alongside the demonisation of slow-release formulated morphine there was an idealisation of methadone, and the clients on methadone maintenance became de-stigmatised. This is ironic, as everything that was said during the campaign to stigmatise slow-release morphine products and their users seems to have been transferred from the stigmatisation of methadone and of methadone clients in the USA. As early as 1974, Miller,[3] summing up the criticisms of methadone maintenance treatment as they are expressed by lobbyists for drug-free treatment, had identified the following points.

- Maintenance treats the symptoms of addiction, not the underlying social and psychological disturbances involved.
- A legal addiction is an unacceptable substitute for an illegal addiction.
- The methadone illusion encourages the nation to assume that human problems can be solved by chemical means.

- Methadone diversion will create a series of street addicts whose primary addiction is to methadone.
- Premature methadone will move individuals on the margins of addiction to a permanent addictive dependence.

In the USA, as a result of these criticisms, methadone treatment has become over-controlled, is prohibited in some localities, and is exposed to strong political influences. Most famous of these is the intervention of New York's Mayor Giuliani, who in 1998 announced the closure of the city's methadone programmes within four years. He assailed the methadone treatment approach as 'immoral' and as merely perpetuating 'enslavement' to narcotics. In 1993, Marc Reisinger stated that in the European Community – following the USA model – methadone treatment had also fallen victim to stigmatisation and had to operate against strong oppositional forces:

> The supply of methadone is inferior to the demand almost everywhere in Europe. This might be seen one day as an unpardonable error of judgement which will cost the lives of hundreds of thousands of persons and wreak havoc on the health care budgets of several European countries.[29]

Ethical problems related to the campaign against slow-release morphine

Since the campaign against the use of slow-release morphine preparations for maintenance purposes utilised the mass media as a communication tool, it has to be seen as having substantial manipulative power. This raises ethical questions, and scare tactics represent a very special problem in this context as they may induce scapegoating and stigmatisation processes, and may even stimulate totalitarian responses.[30,31] The campaign in Austria has proved to be no exception to this. Slow-release morphine preparations became the scapegoat for all known and foreseeable negative side-effects of the medical use of all opioid substances (including methadone). Finally, slow-release morphine preparations themselves became stigmatised, as is illustrated by a campaign leaflet authored by Dr Gross in November 2004:

> The patients are becoming really addicted through these medications (Argument 15).

> Patients treated with high doses of slow-release morphine are not able to work . . . (Argument 8).

> On the black market, slow-release morphine has replaced heroin . . . (Argument 6).

> On the Viennese open drug scene, cocaine abuse increased mark-
> edly. Patients tell that that abuse is financed through the diversion of
> slow-release morphine . . . (Argument 16).

None of these statements were supported by the results of rigorous research. They are based on statements from clients, which were not systematically collected. No recent research data are available with regard to the Viennese drug scene and the illicit market situation.

After the stigmatisation of slow-release morphine had occurred, a process of stigmatisation developed that encroached on drug treatment clients, physicians and the pharmaceutical industry. Certain members of the campaign described clients who were maintained on slow-release morphine preparations as 'drug fiends', bluffing to their doctors to get them to prescribe morphine at elevated dosages, and making their living by diverting a substantial proportion of their prescription to the illicit market. Unemployed clients became a particular target of this labelling. Physicians were described by campaigners as badly educated with regard to the special difficulties that arise from maintenance treatment, and as rather helpless in the face of their clients' guile. As Argument 2 of Dr Gross's campaign leaflet expressed it:

> Slow-release morphine preparations . . . look like Smarties [coloured
> sweets] and are prescribed carelessly by certain physicians . . . How
> shall the general population be aware of the risks when even medical
> doctors are unable to assess them? In school they have been
> cautioned against heroin, but not against slow-release morphine . . .

Physicians were also accused of acting in an irresponsible way, spreading addiction and being 'on the payroll of manufacturers.' The drug-manufacturing industry was not only accused of playing the role of 'legal pusher', but was also blamed for corrupting medical doctors and for contributing to the spread of addictive diseases and their conse-quences. In late 2004, a member of the campaign, Dr Martin Sprenger, circulated a letter that included the following statement:

> Since their introduction in the year 1998, slow-release morphine
> preparations have been pushed on to the Austrian substitution
> market with a massive effort by the drug industry. The prescription
> was left to general practitioners trained by members of pharma-
> ceutical companies.

Impact on the political level

The campaigners gained support from political forces. One example of this is a press conference that was held by the health spokesperson of the FPÖ (the right-wing Freedom Party which is the junior partner in the governing coalition) on 2 February 2005, together with one of the main activists, the above-mentioned Dr Gross. In the context of that event, the prohibition of the use of slow-release formulated morphine was openly suggested. The main argument for that proposal was that heroin addicts are pushed into morphine addiction by the use of morphine preparations for maintenance treatment.

Discussion

Using the history of drug problems and drug control as a system of reference, it can be seen that, in many respects, the campaign against slow-release morphine treatment resembles that against heroin in the USA, which in 1924 prepared the public to accept the prohibition of heroin. In the context of that campaign, heroin was blamed for destroying all sense of moral responsibility, being the drug of the criminal, recruiting its users from young people, and only able to be eliminated by international action. Likewise, in 2005, slow-release morphine has been blamed for recruiting young people as its users, being the drug of choice of unemployed petty criminals who make their living by diverting the substance to the illicit market, and prolonging the career of addiction. Again, international action was stipulated as necessary to eradicate its use. Deconstructing the 1920s campaign against heroin, Trebach[32] pointed out that virtually every 'fact' about the evil of heroin that was testified to under oath was unsupported by any sound evidence, but that nevertheless all misinterpretations went unchallenged. This is comparable to the reaction to the case against slow-release morphine treatment that took place at the political level in Austria.

It is difficult to interpret how the campaign affected Austrian drug policies, but there is no doubt that politicians came under pressure to act, and it may be no coincidence that a change in the government attitude to maintenance treatment can currently be observed, going in exactly the direction desired by the campaigners. At the time of writing, discussions about differentiated regulations and the installation of a rigid control system are under way. Without any further research, an amendment of the Austrian *Suchtgiftverordnung* (the set of regulations that controls the handling of narcotics) has been formulated that subjects the prescribing doctors to elaborate control mechanisms. The draft version of the amendment to the *Suchtgiftverordnung* includes the prohibition of the prescription of preparations containing slow-release morphine. In the discussion that followed the release of this draft, maintenance treatment experts expressed their fears that such a step would destabilise the drug care system that has been developed in Austria, and would endanger the diversification of substances that, for most of those working with maintenance clients, have proved efficient and safe and have been interpreted as a mainstay of the implementation of the harm reduction approach.

The Austrian experience demonstrates the rather fragile 'semi-deviant'[3] status of medication-assisted treatment and the 'marginal identity'[6] of its clients. A certain ambivalence about maintenance treatment can be detected among the general population, since it challenges the concepts and philosophy of a drug-free society. In 1990, Ben-Yehuda[33] demonstrated that methadone treatment is part of a moral debate in which the philosophies of abstinence and maintenance clash. Since the original ideological debate about the nature of addiction has not been resolved, the medicalisation of an addictive disorder is not accepted without reservation. Furthermore, even when opiate addiction is accepted as an illness, there is no consensus about the metabolic theory of addiction and the concept of morphine maintenance treatment. The stigma associated with 'morphine addicts' has also not been resolved. From the history of methadone maintenance treatment, there is a readiness to transfer the stigma of heroin addiction to the maintained state (as in the Guiliani case described above) and to include all concerned parties – doctors, clients and the producers of the medication – in the process of stigmatisation.

In the Austrian case, labelling has shifted from the heroin addict to the client maintained on slow-release morphine, and the stigmatisation has been transferred from heroin addiction to morphine treatment. A specific set of labels has been developed to distinguish the client and the medication, and the status of these clients as medical patients is questioned or even completely denied – they are demonised and presented as representing all the negative characteristics attributed to drug users on the open drug scene. Clearly, the mythological 'drug fiend' described by Lindesmith[34] in 1940 is sleeping in the background and can easily be awakened. Since maintenance treatment using slow-release morphine is considered to be a substitute addiction, it is a special case of tertiary deviance, and people receiving such medication fall within the particular category of stigmatised individuals who, according to Goffmann,[35] include alcoholics, homosexuals, criminals and people with mental disorders. The case against slow-release morphine represents the original cultural ambivalence. It took its power from the attitude that emanates from that ambivalence, and similarly supports it. It will possibly put an end to the Austrian method of diversified medical treatment of opiate dependency.

References

1 Winick C. The deviance model of drug-taking behaviour: a critique. *J Ethnic Cult Diversity Soc Work*. 1986; **1**: 29–49.

2 Young J. *The Drug Takers*. London: Paladin; 1971.

3 Miller R. Towards a sociology of methadone maintenance. In: Winick C, editor. *Sociological Aspects of Drug Dependence*. Cleveland, OH: CRC Press; 1974.

4 Kallen E. *Label Me Human: minority rights of stigmatized Canadians*. Toronto: University of Toronto Press; 1989.

5 Acker CJ. Stigma or legitimation? A historical examination of the social potential of addiction disease models. *J Psychoactive Drugs*. 1993; **25:** 193–205.

6 Murphy S, Irwin J. Living with the dirty secret: problems of disclosure for methadone maintenance clients. *J Psychoactive Drugs*. 1992; **24:** 257–64.

7 Joseph H. *Medical methadone maintenance: the further concealment of a stigmatized condition*. Doctoral thesis, Web version. New York: University of New York, Dora Weiner Foundation; 1995.

8 Kitsuse JI. Coming out all over: deviants and the politics of social problems. *Soc Problems*. 1980; **28:** 1–13.

9 Clinard MB, Meier RF. *Sociology of Deviant Behavior*. 10th ed. Orlando, FL: Harcourt Brace; 1998.

10 European Monitoring Centre for Drugs and Drug Addiction (EMCDDA). *Annual Reports 2000–2003*. Lisbon: EMCDDA.

11 Pompidou Group. *The Multi-City Study*. Strasbourg: Council of Europe Publishing; 1993.

12 Farrell M, Neeleman J, Gossop M *et al*. *A Review of the Legislation, Regulation and Delivery of Methadone in 12 Member States in the European Union*. Brussels: European Commission; 1996.

13 World Health Organization. *European Summary of Drug Abuse. First Report, 1985–1990*. Geneva: World Health Organization Regional Office for Europe; 1992.

14 Gossop M, Grant M. *The Content and Structure of Methadone Treatment Programmes: a study in six countries*. Geneva: World Health Organization, Programme on Substance Abuse; 1990.

15 Nadelmann E, Mcneely J, Drucker E. Harm reduction: international perspectives. In: Lowinson JH, Ruiz P, Millman RB *et al*., editors. *Substance Abuse: a comprehensive textbook*. Baltimore, MD: Williams & Wilkins; 1997.

16 Commonwealth Department of Health and Aged Care. *National Action Plan on Illicit Drugs, 2001–2002-03*. Canberra: Commonwealth Department of Health and Aged Care; 2001.

17 EU Drugs Action Plan, 2005–2008. *Official Journal of the European Union*, 8 July 2005.

18 Springer A. *Different types of medically assisted treatment*. Paper presented at EBDD Meeting on treatment monitoring and the EU Action Plan on Drugs 2000–2004, held at the European Monitoring Centre for Drugs and Drug Addiction, Lisbon, 27–28 November 2003.

19 ÖBIG. *Bericht zur Drogensituation 2004 [Report on the Drug Situation 2004]*. Vienna: Österreichisches Bundesinstitut für Gesundheitswesen; 2004.

20 ÖBIG. *Bericht zur Drogensituation 2003 [Report on the Drug Situation 2003]*. Vienna: Österreichisches Bundesinstitut für Gesundheitswesen; 2003.

21 ÖBIG. *Bericht zur Drogensituation 2005 [Report on the Drug Situation 2005]*. Vienna: Österreichisches Bundesinstitut für Gesundheitswesen; 2005.

22 Uhl A, Springer A, Werner E. *Substitutionstherapie in Österreich (Substitution Treatment in Austria: research report]*. Vienna: Bundesministerium für Gesundheit, Sport und Konsumentenschutz, Forschungsbericht 1; 1992.

23 Haltmayer H, Schmid R. *Untersuchungen über den i.v. Drogenkonsum durch Spritzentests [Research on Intravenous Drug Use by Testing the Residue in Used Syringes]*. Vienna: Forschungsbericht VWS; 2004.

24 Neubauer P, Strobel S. *Drogen-Straßenszene und Substitutionsbehandlung in Wien [The Open Drug Scene and Substitution Treatment in Vienna]*. Vienna: Forschungsbericht VWS; 1998.

25 Fischer G, Jagsch R, Eder H *et al*. Comparison of methadone and slow-release morphine maintenance in pregnant addicts. *Addiction*. 1999; **94**: 231–40.

26 Fischer G, Presslich O, Diamant K *et al*. Oral morphine-sulfate in the treatment of opiate-dependent patients. *Alcoholism*. 1996; **32**: 35–43.

27 Kraigher D, Jagsch R, Wolfgang Gombas W *et al*. Use of slow-release oral morphine for the treatment of opioid dependence. *Eur Addiction Res*. 2005; **11**: 145–51.

28 Mitchell TB, White JM, Somogyi AA *et al*. Slow-release oral morphine versus methadone: a crossover comparison of patient outcomes and acceptability as maintenance pharmacotherapies for opioid dependence. *Addiction*. 2004; **99**: 940–45.

29 Reisinger M, editor. *AIDS and Drug Addiction in the European Community: treatment and mistreatment*. Brussels: European Monitoring Centre for Drugs and Drug Addiction; 1993.

30 Meerloo JAM. *Mental Seduction and Menticide. The psychology of thought control and brainwashing*. London: Jonathan Cape; 1997.

31 Springer A. Drug prevention and the media: conceptualization and some ethical considerations. In: Franke S, Sande M, editors. *Empowering NGOs in Drug Demand Reduction*. Vienna: Care Austria; 2004.

32 Trebach A. *The Heroin Solution*. New Haven, CT: Yale University Press; 1982.

33 Ben-Yehuda N. *The Politics and Morality of Deviance: moral panic, drug abuse and reversed stigmatization*. Albany, NY: State University of New York Press; 1990.

34 Lindesmith AR. Dope fiend mythology. *J Am Inst Crim Law Criminol*. 1940; **31**: 199–208.

35 Goffman E. *Stigma: notes on the management of spoiled identity*. Harmondsworth: Penguin; 1963.

Chapter 9

The methadone game: control strategies and responses

Helle Vibeke Dahl

During my study on the everyday life of methadone maintenance clients in Denmark, it became clear that in addition to the official and medical aims of stabilising and 'normalising' drug addicts, methadone and methadone maintenance treatment serve other important purposes. In this chapter, I will describe how methadone and methadone clinics can be seen as central means of controlling and disciplining drug addicts. I will illustrate how the clients respond to this surveillance and control, and finally I will demonstrate that, in the views and hands of the clients, methadone represents far more than a medical substitute for heroin.

Introduction to the game

When I first introduced the term 'game' into the title of my paper, I was primarily thinking of the 'hide-and-seek' performances that came to my attention during my study. More specifically, I refer to the creative ploys used by the clients (with varying degrees of success) in order to bend the rules and distract and cheat the clinic staff. I must admit that these ploys were not without a certain entertainment value. Nevertheless, both within and outside methadone clinics in Denmark – and elsewhere – a rather serious game is being played. Not only is the history of medical involvement with opiate addiction marked by overt political conflict,[1,2] but also it can be argued that powerful forces are at play, including international and national politics and drug policies, global and local economies, science and scientific approaches and ideology, and morality.[1-5] Re-reading my coded interview transcriptions and fieldnotes, I realised that my initial interpretation of the 'methadone game' could and should be expanded to include attention to the influence of the forces of global and national players or rule makers on the lives of methadone clients.

My informants quite often used the game metaphor when describing their situation and perspectives. One of them was Paul, a long-term methadone client in his forties. Paul always became very animated when talking about methadone and especially the clinic where he collected his methadone once a week. For example:

> Life is a game, that's what my old man always told us . . . and I'm well aware that I'm only a pawn in the game, but that doesn't mean that I play the way they want us to in the clinic. If I had stuck to their rules, I would have been in prison or dead by now – or been turned into one of these zombies you see around here [at the clinic].

A little later in the interview, he dismissed one of my arguments by insisting that I still hadn't grasped 'what it's all about':

> If you really want to write about how it is to be one of us, you'll have to realise that it has less to do with drugs or medicine, and everything to do with the way we are treated by society, by the systems that are supposed to help us, by . . . [pausing, then raising his voice] It is one big fucking game, can't you see? It's big money, it's drugs and weapons and financing wars and it's the whole fucking drug industry, it's the insurance companies and all you people in the treatment systems and research whatever . . . it's everybody . . . Yeah, everybody plays their game and so do I, but in the eyes of society we are already losers. And honestly, I think they are quite satisfied that we are drug addicts, because they know how we can be pacified, doped to pieces by methadone and pills prescribed by the state. 'Dope them, man, dope them – and they'll shut up!' That's how they think . . .

The lives of those who are dependent on illicit drugs can be harsh and strenuous, but what is less well recognised is that life on a methadone maintenance programme also has its darker side, as the treatment does not automatically rehabilitate the client. Both in the eyes of society and in their own experience, as indicated by Paul, methadone maintenance clients are regarded as outsiders and social inferiors, and are thus marginalised and stigmatised. Individuals who have been marginalised socially, economically and culturally are likely to develop a negative long-term relationship with mainstream society.[4,6] For Paul and many others in a similar situation, the experience of being 'a pawn in the game' can be interpreted as a consequence of this negative long-term relationship, but it may also be a reflection or consequence of society's ambivalence towards methadone maintenance: 'being a methadone patient is a marginal identity; not quite junkie, not quite conventional.'[7] The experiences of such marginalised individuals and their responses to those experiences are the central issues that will be addressed in this chapter.

Aim and research methods

The specific aim of this chapter is to describe how the methadone game manifests itself locally. A more general aim is to illustrate how methadone maintenance and methadone clients are perceived in the research literature, and to discuss the status and expansion of methadone maintenance treatment in this context. I shall summarise the history of methadone maintenance and the role that it has played – and is supposed to play – in relation to opiate addiction, then I shall present the strategies and perspectives of the main players and actors in one specific clinic setting, and finally I shall discuss the roles that methadone plays in the lives of clients by illustrating why and how the game is initiated.

During my study, clinics that varied in type, size and operation served as central sites for building relationships and making observations. Data have primarily been gathered during one year of intensive ethnographic fieldwork in four methadone clinics, open street drug scenes, low threshold facilities and regular visits to a prison ward for female inmates in drug treatment. In the tradition of ethnographic fieldwork, the main data production methods were qualitative interviews and participant observation, including the often painstaking and time-consuming task of writing fieldnotes (of observations, impressions, conversations, reflections, preliminary analyses, etc.).[8] The resulting several hundred pages of data were coded in the computer-based software program NVivo 2.0, as were 10 semi-structured interviews with clinic doctors and staff and 40 semi-structured and open-ended life-story interviews with men and women who had been receiving methadone maintenance treatment for up to 30 years.

The predominant methodological approach in the research on drug treatment has been quantitative, with qualitative studies playing only a minor or marginal role.[3,5,9] Focusing on the practice and rules in a specific methadone setting, my primary aim has been to capture the view and voice of the clients, who in the bulk of the research literature on drug treatment, including methadone therapy, have been systematically reduced to objects to be controlled and measured:

> They are, in effect, transformed into passive figures on to which a treatment modality is applied. Their social identity is reduced to a set of demographic characteristics, such as age, gender and ethnicity, which may or may not bear on the success of the treatment.[10]

Since the 1960s, several (mostly American) ethnographic and other qualitative studies have focused on the attitudes, experiences and perceptions of drug users, producing an altogether different picture in which the users, whether in or out of treatment, are acting rationally and strategically.[7,10–13] In addition, qualitative research methodologies and approaches have been a central means of describing the influence and interplay of individual, social and contextual factors (such as historical, cultural and economic contexts) with regard to drug use and treatment.[4,14–17]

The history of methadone and the institutionalisation of methadone maintenance

The history of drug addiction includes the history of the search for a medical cure for it. Examples of so-called miracle or therapeutic cures are plentiful. In the late eighteenth century, morphine was believed to cure cocaine addiction, injected morphine was used to cure opium addiction, and heroin was explicitly marketed as a non-addictive cure for morphine addiction.[1,18] In the 1930s, a series of new synthetic analgesics were marketed and accepted as safe and curative, including what is now known as methadone, an opiate-like drug synthesised in Germany during the Second World War, and commercially produced under many different trade names from 1947.[19] Although mainly prescribed for its pain-killing properties, methadone was also used for detoxification purposes.[20,21] However, it was not until the mid-1960s that it was discovered to be an effective medical substitute for illicit opioids. Vincent Dole and Marie Nyswander had found that when it was administered orally and in an adequate dose, the pharmacological effects of methadone would prevent withdrawal symptoms for 24–36 hours, relieve drug craving and block the euphoric effects of heroin.[22] Significantly, the results of Dole and Nyswander's pioneering study indicated that when stabilised on methadone, their patients were able to reorganise their lives socially and productively. Since then, treatment with methadone has expanded substantially to become the predominant form of drug treatment in most western countries.[23,24]

Methadone prescribing in Denmark

In the mid-1960s, Denmark was the first country outside the USA to introduce a methadone maintenance programme.[25] Although the early results of the Danish programme were far from convincing,[26] and despite the fact that methadone maintenance has been a much debated issue ever since, it has expanded to become the main drug treatment modality in Denmark. During the period 1985–2003, the number of people receiving methadone maintenance treatment (defined by the National Health Board as treatment for more than five months) increased from 897 to 5,229.[27]

The organisation and delivery of methadone programmes vary both between and within countries,[23] and despite a reform in 1996 to centralise and standardise drug treatment services in general, Danish methadone maintenance programmes show major variations both between and within regions. The most important variations can be defined in terms of control policy (how the head of a clinic interprets Denmark's guidelines), such as how strictly clients' intake of methadone and their urine samples are supervised, the consequences of supplementary drug use, and 'take-home' policies. There may also be variation in opening hours, dosage policies, and whether psychosocial treatment services are an integrated part of the clinic's programme. Despite these variations, the majority of the research sample consistently reported a strained relationship with the system on which their maintenance arrangements depended, and a strong wish for self-management. However, as will be discussed below, regardless of whether the programmes have a liberal or restrictive control policy, the methadone that is dispensed serves more than its prescribed purposes.

Treatment effectiveness and perspectives as game factors

Methadone maintenance treatment is the most thoroughly evaluated intervention in the field of drug addiction. During the last 40 years, numerous international, medical and quantitative research studies and evaluations have almost ritually reported the effectiveness of the treatment, particularly in reducing heroin use, injecting and criminal activity.[28] With methadone as the chemical agent, drug users have been given the opportunity – and are expected – to stop using illegal drugs and injecting, improve their health and stabilise and reorganise their lives. While Danish research has demonstrated similar outcomes to those of studies conducted elsewhere, the results have also concurred with the findings of other studies that a reduction in the use of illegal opiates and criminal activity does not automatically result in physical, psychological and social improvements in the lives of the clients.[29,30] For example, a recently published review criticised traditional and biomedical evaluation approaches for highlighting the 'successes' of methadone maintenance and downplaying the evidence of severe limitations, including the fact that 'focusing on a patient-centred perception of health and well-being has played a completely marginal role.'[31] It is tempting to conclude that these shortcomings have been the reason why methadone and methadone maintenance have continually been an ambivalent and controversial issue, both politically and among professionals. However, they may importantly indicate that the health and well-being of methadone clients is of minor importance and subordinated to societal measures of 'success':

> . . . it must be emphasized that methadone maintenance did not expand because society wanted to provide treatment for heroin

addicts. On the contrary, the main concern was reducing the number of crimes committed by addicts. That included the curtailment of the spread of addiction-related infections such as HIV and hepatitis.[24]

In his research on methadone treatment, the Danish anthropologist Steffen Jöhncke has studied the way that drug users are made into objects of policy and subjects of treatment, and how acts of oppression take place 'in the hidden details of bureaucratic and political practice.'[32] According to his perception, treatment is not simply an institutional practice, but also an indication of cultural values, such as how 'good' we as a society perceive ourselves to be:

> Practices of drug use and practices of treatment are constructed as moral opposites, the unconditionally evil countered by the unconditionally good – forming an interlocking, moral whole against which objections are unthinkable. In this perspective, for all the positive effects treatment might also provide, it is also part of a system of social welfare practices that construct the drug user as antithetical to what it means to be a proper person in contemporary Denmark. [32]

From this perspective, to analyse treatment practices simply as benevolent and humanistic enterprises not only obscures the game of power, but also disguises the multifaceted ways in which power operates in order to control and discipline the clients.[32–34]

The controversial status of methadone maintenance treatment is primarily an outcome of the pharmacological qualities of methadone, which soon proved to be just as addictive as heroin (some claim even more so). Thus methadone maintenance has been defined by critics as prolonging addiction and/or rejected on the grounds that it simply replaced one drug (illegal heroin) with another (legally prescribed methadone).[1,35] In short, methadone is an emotionally charged, politically sensitive issue. To maintain drug users on a potent and addictive drug is at odds with the abstinence-oriented ideology that dominates most national drug treatment policies, and the risk of diversion to the illicit market has been a prominent concern. Consequently, methadone maintenance has come to represent a rather unique treatment modality in which one of the dominant characteristics is the extensive spectrum of strategies for controlling the dispensed drug and its users.

However, despite great efforts to ensure that the methadone ends up in the right bodies and in the prescribed way and dose, the drug is employed for a variety of purposes that go beyond purely medical ones. Thus we arrive at the clinic where I 'hung out' for almost six months with the aim of documenting the experiences, perceptions, values and actions of the individuals involved.

The local playing field

In a quiet street in the city centre, a discreet sign announces 'County centre.' The methadone clinic has around 350 clients, but its physical setting is relatively small. The low clinic building is anonymous, standing back from the other houses and with a lawn in front of it. Although the area is deserted after noon, it is quite busy during the morning hours, with people coming, going or lingering.

What strikes you when you enter the clinic's reception room is the tall wooden counter that physically separates the clinic staff from the clients. Except for a few posters on the walls and a couple of café tables and chairs, the room is almost bare, and the metal bench in front of the dispensing counter is uninviting. On each side of the counter, two permanently locked doors lead to the staff and clinic doctor's offices and the toilets. During opening hours, the clients queue up in front of the counter to be served their medicine, make appointments to see the clinic doctor, and so on. Usually four clinic employees are present behind the counter, busy attending to the administration and dispensing of methadone and other types of medicine prepared for each client.

Of the 350 clients who were enrolled at this methadone clinic at the time of the study, around 125 collected their dose of methadone every day, including those who were enrolled on the programme for the purpose of a short detoxification. The majority of the individuals in this group were considered unable to administer take-home doses, typically because they were still using an often substantial amount of illegal drugs, but also because their use of alcohol was regarded as problematic. A further 125 clients collected their methadone every two or three days. This group consisted of a mixed category of clients, half of them striving to prove that they merited the privilege of being trusted with a take-home weekly ration, and the other half striving to keep their current arrangement. The remaining 100 clients were given their doses once a week. They were considered to be the most stabilised and well-functioning clients.

Medical rationales and control strategies

Being a drug clinic doctor does not appear to be a particularly attractive option, as one of three posts at the clinic had been vacant for over a year. However, this did not affect the great enthusiasm for methadone maintenance of the two doctors in charge:

> Listen! Medical drug abuse treatment is provided to secure a stable, daily intake of medicine, because the receptors in the brain must be saturated. If not provided [with medicine] they will go up and down between euphoria and withdrawal, euphoria and withdrawal. And

that's what drives you into a silly behaviour and way of living. But with the stable and daily intake of medicine we provide from here, your central nervous system will calm down, and then you will get the opportunity to do something about all the other problems.

Until five or six years ago, supplementary drug use by a client on the methadone maintenance programme would typically result in a transfer to a rapidly reducing detoxification programme, but today 'a more harm-reduction-oriented attitude' prevails, which according to one of the doctors is much more humane:

> The control is the same but our responses to what we detect are different . . . what we do is this. We pull people into the office: 'What is happening? What can we do for you? Do you need more methadone? What about residential treatment to reduce your drug abuse?' And so on. We are absolutely no longer interested in throwing people back on to the streets. Oh no!

The staff explained the regular control elements used at the clinic by emphasising that the supervised administration of methadone mixture, breath tests and random urine tests delivered under surveillance must be seen as security measures for the sake of the clients:

> Our job is to provide the proper and safe medical treatment, see to the well-being and health of the patients, and prevent them from killing themselves while they are in our treatment.

According to the clinic policy, the clients may, after an initial phase during which they are expected to stabilise medically and functionally, be allowed to take their doses home, typically starting with a weekend's ration. According to one of the doctors, the two principal criteria for deciding whether a client can be trusted with take-home doses are 'their conduct', meaning 'acceptable and compliant behaviour', and 'their ability to provide clean urine samples' over an unspecified period of time.

User perspectives and responses to the clinic setting

Heroin and polydrug users may have multiple motives for entering methadone maintenance programmes, whether short- or long-term. The primary reasons cited by my informants demonstrate that methadone is seen as a means of freeing themselves completely from illicit drug dependence, or of decreasing their use of illegal drugs in order to get their habit under control and/or reduce the risks accompanying it.

Despite the pharmacological properties of methadone (blocking the euphoric effects of heroin and suppressing cravings for opiates), according to a recent study on 422 drug users from the three main cities of Denmark,[29] only a few methadone clients stop using illegal drugs altogether. The data from my study confirm this conclusion, and from a user's perspective it is unsurprising:

> The problem is that society will not understand that drug users use drugs, we are used to doping ourselves whatever our individual reasons may be, and it doesn't just stop because of a dose of methadone.

However, the continued use of illegal drugs does not mean that methadone is rendered superfluous. My informants typically emphasised that methadone had minimised their use of illegal drugs and to some extent stabilised their life situation. However, they also revealed a darker side to the picture:

> Methadone keeps you from being sick, that's true, but you really get dependent on that drug and, what's worse, you are dependent on the system and all the things that follow, all their demands and rules. You lose your freedom and if you are not strong you lose your self-respect.

As described above, the main reward for adhering to the clinic's regulations is being entrusted with up to a week's supply of methadone for unsupervised self-administration. Whatever their individual arrangements with regard to take-home supplies, the clinic nevertheless attracted very negative comments from the majority of the clients. This general discontent centred primarily on being dependent on the clinic, the limited opening hours, and especially the surveillance and measures of control that accompany the methadone maintenance programme.

The motives for obtaining take-home doses were many and varied, and a few are given here as examples. One centred around a dislike of visiting the clinic. Every day, clients would congregate outside the clinic in small groups, talking, smoking and drinking strong beer. Some of the other clients found it intimidating to pass these groups, and likened it to 'running the gauntlet.' In addition, as one client pointed out, 'It is one thing to pass this crowd. Another is the temptations you are exposed to, and I'm a weak person when it comes to that.' These temptations include not only the drugs that are offered for sale, but also the inclination to stay on, socialise and eventually use illicit drugs, buy some beer, and so on. Female clients in particular expressed their dislike of and unease about entering and leaving the clinic because of the transactions, hustling, and frequent episodes of violence and theft.

Another reason why clients disliked the clinic was because they had to queue up in front of the dispensing counter. At times, around 10 to 15 people were in the queue, and the lack of patience could result in verbal and physical aggression. Despite the advice from the staff to compare it to queuing in the supermarket or the bank, many clients expressed the view that the practice evoked feelings of being exposed and humiliated:

> I just hate standing in that line, it's so shameful. We are like cattle waiting to be watered. And when you reach the counter they ask 'Name?' I don't want everyone around me to know my name, and I find it embarrassing to be watched when I drink my methadone. And when they ask me to go and give a urine test before they pass my methadone . . . oh, it's so humiliating! In their eyes we are nothing but a bunch of lousy junkies – no respect is shown.

A central aspiration of clients was to be in possession and control of the methadone itself. Apart from its role as medicine, methadone is an attractive and valuable object. It serves as a drug that some clients prefer because of its mild but pleasant and long-lasting euphoria, or it can be used as a base drug to be boosted with alcohol or other drugs.[36,37] Methadone is easy to sell and can be exchanged for other drugs and goods,[38] and is therefore viewed as a useful addition to a poor economy. Methadone is also circulated among friends as a loan or gift, and from this perspective the drug has important functions in social bonding. Lending or giving away methadone to friends or potential friends is a way to create and maintain social relationships, and serves as insurance for reciprocation. Thus, in the hands of the clients, methadone represents both economic and social security.

Despite medical advice and clinic rules – and sanctions if disclosed – clients with take-home doses were likely to develop their own self-maintenance programmes. The individual models varied widely, and included the following. According to the medical prescription, the daily methadone dose must be taken once a day. However, many clients preferred to divide the daily dose into two or three smaller doses, in some cases because they became too drowsy and passive for a couple of hours after taking it all, and in others because they experienced withdrawal symptoms towards the end of the 24 hours. However, these self-regulation patterns were disrupted when clients visited the clinic for fresh take-home supplies, because on that day the full dose had to be swallowed under supervision. From the clients' point of view, this rule was incomprehensible and contrary to their experiences of well-being. Consequently, in order to avoid having to consume more than usual, it was not uncommon for them to try to leave the clinic with their cup of methadone hidden in their pocket or up their sleeve, to spill some of the methadone liquid on to the floor or in the wastepaper basket, or to share their dose with another client in exchange for an empty cup.

Many of the methadone clients tried to manage their dependence on the drug by reducing or increasing their prescribed dose. On occasion, for example, some clients reduced their methadone intake in order to get a good 'high' from heroin. From a medical perspective, these strategies were viewed as both irresponsible and counterproductive and, if discovered, the client would be required to attend the clinic for daily supervised methadone consumption.

One of the unwritten rules of the clinic was 'In order for us to help you, you've got to be honest.' However, in the experience of the clients, honesty more often than not had undesirable consequences. For example, if before a urine test a client tells the clinic staff that they will test positive because they have used heroin or cocaine once, and the result is that the take-home methadone arrangement is withdrawn, clients will not see this as helpful, but rather as a punishment. Next time, in the same situation, they will therefore try to avoid the test or cheat it. Another example involved a client who confessed that she had taken extra methadone and would run out of supplies before she received her next take-home supply. As a result, she was deemed unfit for self-administration, and she made the following comment:

> You only make that mistake once, and then they can talk as much about honesty as they want. In this system honesty is risky business. Forget it.

Experiences like this generate and support secrecy and lies, and encourage clients to play a dishonest game. However, it was not uncommon for clients to admit that the faking strategies could be difficult to maintain in times of trouble. For example:

> They see me as a model client. They never had a thing on me. Nothing at all! They even don't know anything about my drinking and my problems with the methadone – I'm careful. But it hits back on me now, because it's getting out of hand. I wish I could trust them. I tell you much more than I would ever tell them.

An experienced methadone client commented indirectly on this issue by stating that the system of methadone maintenance keeps the clients fixed in their identity as drug addicts and untrustworthy deviants. After more than 15 years in maintenance treatment, he believed that he had finally learned to play the game:

> But you have to be smart to play the game and to get things the way you want, or at least in a way that makes you feel that you're still in some control. Just take a look around . . . many of these guys lining up in the queue, they are just not smart enough, they have to come to pick up their dose every single day and they have done so for years. They are stuck . . . and that's not to say that I'm better than they are, I'm a drug addict as well. I was actually convinced that heroin would be my drug for ever, but luckily methadone has become my favourite. In addition . . . it's free and it [extra doses] doesn't show in the urine.

So what is at stake in this game? Conclusion

During the last 40 years, numerous quantitative studies have demon-strated the effectiveness of methadone maintenance treatment, but qual-itative studies that include the opinions and experiences of the clients render the picture blurred and ambiguous. In this chapter, methadone maintenance treatment has been illuminated from different angles and from different individuals' perspectives, revealing a considerable gap between the treatment ideals and practices of the medical professionals and the way in which these are perceived and experienced by clients. The main issue at stake can be summed up in one word – 'control.'

Control operates at several levels and with various aims. In summary, from a political and societal point of view, drug addicts represent criminal and social disorder, and the state's two main responses are punishment and drug treatment services. In the view of the medical profession, drug addiction is a disease to be treated medically, and methadone maintenance treatment has become the primary response. However, the treatment of drug addiction with methadone depends on government policy. Consequently, the adoption of methadone mainten-ance treatment places medicine and the methadone doctor in the service of the government, 'with medicine functioning as a social control agent for the state.'[1] At the clinic level, the control elements and strategies employed therefore have a double goal – the purely medical control exerted in order to assess the effectiveness of the treatment, and the state's control exerted in order to prevent diversion.

However, from the client's perspective, the control regime of the methadone clinic is perceived as yet another reminder of their inferior and marginalised status. If they are confronted with a restrictive and supervised clinic setting, methadone is likely to become a means of upholding or gaining (self-)control and (self-)respect, and of maintaining what Klein has called 'autonomy over their pharmacological state.'[2]

References

1 Conrad P, Schneider JW. *Deviance and Medicalization. From badness to sickness.* 2nd ed. Philadelphia, PA: Temple University Press; 1992.
2 Klein D. Ill and against the law: the social control and medical control of heroin users. *J Drug Issues.* 1983; **133**: 31–55.
3 Agar M. How the drug field turned my beard grey. *Int J Drug Policy.* 2002; **13**: 249–58.
4 Bourgois P. *In Search of Respect: selling crack in El Barrio.* New York: Cambridge University Press.1995.
5 Bourgois P, Lettiere M, Quesada J. Social misery and the sanctions of substance abuse: confronting HIV risk among homeless heroin addicts in San Francisco. *Soc Problems.* 1997; **44**: 155–73.

6 Merton RK. *Social Theory and Social Structure*. New York: The Free Press; 1968.
7 Murphy S, Irwin J. 'Living with the dirty secret': problems of disclosure for methadone maintenance clients. *J Psychoactive Drugs*. 1992; **24**: 257–64.
8 Emerson RM, Fretz RI, Shaw LL. *Writing Ethnographic Fieldnotes*. Chicago: University of Chicago Press; 1995.
9 Rhodes T. The multiple roles of qualitative research in understanding and responding to illicit drug use. In: *Understanding and Responding to Drug Use: the role of qualitative research*. EMCDDA Scientific Monograph. Lisbon: European Monitoring Centre for Drugs and Drug Addiction (EMCDDA); 2000.
10 Hunt G, Rosenbaum M. 'Hustling' within the clinic: consumer perspectives on methadone maintenance treatment. In: Inciardi JA, Harrison LD, editors. *Heroin in the Age of Crack-Cocaine*. Thousands Oaks, CA: Sage Publications; 1998.
11 Preble E, Casey JJ. Taking care of business – the heroin user's life on the street. *Int J Addiction*. 1969; **4**: 1–24.
12 Rosenbaum M. *Women on Heroin*. New Brunswick: Rutgers University Press; 1981.
13 Koester S, Anderson K, Hoffer L. Active heroin injectors' perceptions and use of methadone maintenance treatment. *Subst Use Misuse*. 1999; **34**: 2135–53.
14 Grund JP. *Drug Use as a Social Ritual: functionality, symbolism and determinants of self-regulation*. Rotterdam: Instituut voor Verslavingsonderzoek; 1993.
15 Taylor A. *Women Drug Users. An ethnography of a female injecting community*. Oxford: Clarendon Press; 1993.
16 Svensson B. *Pundare, Jonkare och Andra [Amphetamine and Heroin Injectors and Others]*. Stockholm: Carlssons; 1996.
17 Dahl HV. Ilde hørt? Den larmende tavshed omkring etnografiske rusmiddelforskning [Unwelcome messages? The noisy silence of ethnographic drug research]. In: Asmussen V, Jöhncke S, editors. *Brugerperspektiver. Fra stofmisbrug til socialpolitik [User Perspectives. From drug misuse to social policy]*. Aarhus: Aarhus Universitetsforlag; 2004.
18 Gossop M. *Living with Drugs*. 5th ed. Aldershot: Ashgate; 2000.
19 Gerlach R. A brief overview on the discovery of methadone; www.indro-online/de/discovery.pdf
20 Isbell H, Vogel VH. The addiction liability of methadone (amidone, dolphine, 10820) and its use in the treatment of the morphine abstinence syndrome. *Am J Psychiatry*. 1949; **195**: 909–14.
21 Nimb M. *Misbrug af Euforiserende Stoffer i Danmark i 1950erne med Efterundersøgelse i 1972 [Abuse of Euphoriants in Denmark in the 1950s with Follow-Up in 1972]*. Aarhus: Villadsen & Christensen; 1975.
22 Dole VP, Nyswander M. A medical treatment for diacetylmorphine (heroin) addiction. *JAMA*. 1965; **193**: 646–50.
23 Farrell M, Ward J, Mattick R *et al*. Methadone maintenance treatment in opiate dependence: a review. *BMJ*. 1994; **30**: 997–1001.
24 Joseph H. Methadone maintenance treatment and clinical issues; www.methadone.org/library/joseph_1994_methadone_clinical.html
25 Jourdan M. Metadonbehandlingens ukendte foregangsmand [The unknown pioneer of methadone treatment]. *STOF*. 2003; **2**: 53–62.
26 Nimb M. *Behandling af narkomaner med vedligeholdelsesdoser af metadon [Treating drug addicts with methadone maintenance doses]*. Unpublished paper from a lecture to the Danish Psychiatric Society, Copenhagen; 13 October 1969.
27 Reitox National Focal Point. *New Developments, Trends and In-Depth Information on Selected Issues. Denmark. National report to the EMCCDA*. Copenhagen: Reitox National Focal Point; 2004.

28 Joseph H, Stancliff S, Langrod J. Methadone maintenance treatment (MMT): a review of historical and clinical issues. *Mt Sinai Med J.* 2000; **67**: 347–64.

29 Pedersen MU. *Substitutionsbehandling. Organiseringer, stofmisbrugere, effekter og metoder [Substitution Treatment. Organisations, drug abusers, effects and methods].* Aarhus: Center for Rusmiddelforskning, University of Aarhus; 2001.

30 Pedersen MU. *Heroin-Afhængige i Metadonbehandling. Den medicinske og psyko-sociale indsats [Heroin Addicts in Methadone Treatment. The medical and psycho-social intervention].* Aarhus: Center for Rusmiddelforskning, University of Aarhus; 2005.

31 Fischer B, Rehm J, Kim G *et al.* Eyes wide shut? A conceptual and empirical critique of methadone maintenance treatment. *Eur Addict Res.* 2005; **11**: 1–14.

32 Jöhncke S. Fieldwork, oppression, and the harsh realities of bureaucratic life. Paper for the Young Scholars' Forum, presented at the Seventh Biennial European Association of Social Anthropologists Conference, Copenhagen, 16 August 2002.

33 Bourgois P. Disciplining addictions: the bio-politics of methadone and heroin in the United States. *Cult Med Psychiatry.* 2000; **24**: 165–95.

34 Bergschmidt VB. Pleasure, power and dangerous substances: applying Foucault to the study of 'heroin dependence' in Germany. *Anthropol Med.* 2004; **11**: 59–73.

35 Ege P. *Stofmisbrug. Baggrund, konsekvenser, behandling [Drug Abuse. Background, consequences, treatment].* Copenhagen: Hans Reitzels Forlag; 1997.

36 Weppner RS, Stephens RC, Contad HT. Methadone: some aspects of its legal and illegal use. *Am J Psychiatry.* 1972; **129**: 451–5.

37 Agar M. The methadone street scene: the addict's view. *Psychiatry.* 1975; **38**: 381–7.

38 Fountain J, Griffiths P, Farrell M *et al.* Diversion tactics: how a sample of drug misusers in treatment obtained surplus drugs to sell on the illicit market. *Int J Drug Pol.* 1998; **9**: 159–67.

Chapter 10

How to camouflage ethical questions in addiction research

Alfred Uhl

> As long as thinking is enjoyable it has not yet started.
>
> Deschner[1]

Policy research is commonly presented as a value-free endeavour but, logically speaking, practical conclusions cannot be derived solely from facts. In research methodology, to attempt to do so is termed the 'Naturalistic Fallacy.' Consequently, the term 'evidence-based policy' – if interpreted literally – constitutes a contradiction in itself (oxymoron). This chapter will also deal with several other fallacies that are encountered in empirical addiction research, will reveal some popular concepts to be inconsistent and illogical advocacy tools, and will argue that the specific role of a researcher is completely incompatible with the role of an advocate for certain ideas and/or interest groups.

The aim of the chapter is to describe and analyse some common logical fallacies in addiction research – particularly some fallacies that camouflage ethical questions – illustrated by some simple examples. I shall not distinguish between fallacies where the perpetrators were victims of their own inadequacy (paralogism) and situations where others were misled on purpose (sophisms), as I am convinced that error and deception are not two distinct categories, but two extremes, with most cases located on the continuum between them. Psychoanalysis tells us that human motives are rarely fully conscious, and dissonance theory tells us that it often easier to deceive oneself than to deliberately deceive others – at least in the long term. Many of the fallacies and the related practical examples discussed here are not difficult for researchers to understand, and have been well known for a long time among methodologists and epistemologists. The following examples are a rather unsystematic selection of unusual perspectives, descriptions of logical flaws and elaborations on methodological problems, put forward to enhance thinking both along critical methodological lines and about the ethical basis behind practical conclusions.

Professionalism – or the 'Wishful Thinking Fallacy'

A few years ago, I gave a lecture on research problems to preventionists and therapists, and a renowned researcher sitting with me on the podium remarked loudly 'I know you are right, but you must not discuss such matters openly in front of these people!' He was even more upset when he realised that his remarks had been heard by the very audience whose trust in science he did not want to jeopardise. This behaviour, located some-where between wishful thinking[2]* on the one hand and deliberately withholding elements of truth for the sake of professionalism on the other, makes it difficult to address uncertainties, ambiguities in termin-ology, empirical and logical contradictions, and value conflicts. Col-leagues undermining a professional reputation by asking nasty questions and putting the finger on weak spots are not welcomed as individuals trying to advance research, but rather are rejected as defeatists working against their own interests. However, this position is very short-sighted. Creating the unrealistic myth that every task can be accomplished puts those who nourish this myth and their colleagues under pressure to achieve impossible tasks. Systematically camouflaging problems allows them to pile up unsolved, until eventually the flawed constructions are uncovered and the reputation of the whole profession is diminished.

Values, ethics and the 'Naturalistic Fallacy'

Statements can be dichotomised into descriptive statements (factual judgements about what is) and prescriptive statements (value judgements about what ought to be done). The latter are referred to as ethical judgements. It is well accepted in philosophy (Hume's Law†) that ethical judgements cannot be derived logically from empirical facts alone.[3] Any syllogism to arrive at ethical conclusions requires at least one ethical premise as well. The flawed idea of basing ethical conclusions purely on empirical facts was called the 'Naturalistic Fallacy' by Moore,[4]‡ and has become a well-known term in research methodology. On the basis of facts, only factual conclusions can be derived. However, this does not

---

* The 'Wishful Thinking Fallacy' refers to rejecting something solely due to wishing that it were not true.
† Hume: 'Reason has no influence on our passions and action. It is in vain to pretend that morality is discovered only by a deduction of reason.'
‡ Moore: 'But if he confuses good, which is not in the same sense a natural object, with any natural object whatever, then there is a reason for calling that a naturalistic fallacy.'

mean that ethical issues cannot be a topic for empirical research – the opposite is true. It is essential to identify implicit value judgements and to make them explicit. Only if all implicit value judgements in our scientific reasoning are made explicit is it possible to analyse whether the ethical premises are consistent with each other,* with basic ethical principles and with factual evidence.† I have previously termed the process of identifying and analysing implicit values in research 'ethical evaluation',[5] but this term is ambiguous since it could mean either 'to conduct evaluations according to ethical standards' or 'to evaluate the ethical content in research.' More precise is the term 'evaluation of implicit ethics' or the almost synonymous 'evaluation of implicit values.'

Evidence-based policy

If we look into the history of medicine and other human sciences and consider how many researchers continue to aggregate questionable research findings, common-sense assumptions and wild speculations into conclusions that are then presented as solid scientific facts, it undoubtedly makes sense to demand that research should be 'evidence based', in the sense of 'conscientious, explicit, and judicious use of current best evidence', as defined by Sackett.[6] However, we must be aware that in most fields of human and social sciences our conclusions – even if we do our best – will remain somewhat uncertain and ambiguous. In most areas, decisive studies in the sense of well-designed, randomised, controlled trials (RCTs) are far beyond reach. As Hartnoll[7] put it, we have to understand research as

> a process where relevant questions evolve, where existing evidence is put together as in a puzzle, where missing pieces are temporarily added based on common sense and logic, and eventually clarified through further research. A researcher, according to this conception, is like a detective who systematically collects and assembles evidence until the case is solved.

If we understand the term 'evidence-based' as Sackett defines it and, in line with Hartnoll's concept of research, if we accept that practical strategies require decisions about ethical principles as well, there is absolutely no objection to the term – but this is not the way that the term 'evidence-based' is commonly used and interpreted. Usually the term carries an aura of 'independence from subjective values' and

---

* For example, the ethical principle of offering the best treatment available to patients is sometimes in conflict with the ethical principle that mature and sane individuals have a right to reject treatment that they do not believe in.
† For example, the ethical principle of offering the best treatment available to patients requires a knowledge of what is the best available treatment.

'proven beyond doubt', which is doubtless inadequate and misleading. The term 'evidence-based policy', if understood as derived solely from evidence, is a contradiction in itself – a 'Natural Fallacy' related to the value-free science myth. The impression of 'proven beyond doubt' is equally unacceptable. To print 'evidence-based' on the covers of medical books like a seal of quality – a popular fashion – is a good example of what Pirie[8] called the 'Fallacy of Blinding with Science.' The notion that authors believe their work makes optimal use of logic and empirical evidence is certainly not new, but until the term 'evidence-based' was coined, declaring this openly was considered arrogant and conceited. Using this new terminology, this presumptuousness can now be presented as a neutral commitment to a specific methodological direction.

Proposed alcohol control policy and the 'Naturalistic Fallacy'

In terms of alcohol control policy, it is important to realise that there are two very distinct perspectives concerning alcohol use in the western world. One perspective is that of the Northern European and Anglo-Saxon 'ambivalence cultures', in contrast to the attitudes in Alpine and Southern European 'tolerance cultures', as Pittman[9]* expressed it. The traditional approach to alcohol in the ambivalence cultures is 'paternalistic/controlling.' The traditional attitude towards alcohol in tolerance cultures is to discriminate strictly between moderate alcohol consumption, as a cultural value and source of pleasure, and alcohol abuse and addiction as problem areas. Consequently, the preferred intervention strategy from the tolerance position is 'democratic/emancipatory', in line with the health promotion concept defined by the World Health Organization (WHO) *Ottawa Charter*.[10] The latter concept does not aim at restricting responsible alcohol use, but rather to reduce the factors influencing transition from responsible use towards problematic use and addiction.

The most important current book in the alcohol policy context is *Alcohol, No Ordinary Commodity* by Babor *et al.*,[11] the third in a series of WHO-sponsored publications, written by alcohol researchers from countries with ambivalence cultures. Since ambivalence cultures had perceived alcohol as a major problem for many decades, they invested much money in alcohol research, while the tolerance cultures did not. As a result, there are now many highly distinguished alcohol researchers from an ambivalence culture background, and hardly any to counterbalance them from a tolerance culture perspective.

---

* Pittman, in relation to alcohol use, discriminated between 'abstinent cultures', 'ambivalent cultures', 'permissive cultures' and 'over-permissive cultures.'

To avoid any misunderstanding, let it be said that *Alcohol, No Ordinary Commodity* was written by some of the most distinguished researchers in the alcohol policy field. It gives a good overview of the relevant empirical literature, in most parts it analyses contradictions and ambiguities within this field of research quite realistically, and it admits that the results are far less consistent and conclusive than one would desire. It can without question be accepted as a standard reference work in the field. On the other hand, the book is clearly written from the perspective of the ambivalence cultures involved, and the summary conclusions do not point out the uncertainties, contradictions and ambiguities mentioned in the main text. The authors reach very clear-cut conclusions, insinuating a degree of validity and reliability that is not at all justified by the overview of research evidence. Their recommendations thus do not confuse those politicians and decision makers who only read summaries and who prefer simple and unequivocal conclusions. This makes the book a useful advocacy tool for activists in favour of the traditional paternalistic alcohol control strategies of Northern Europe, and an almost unchallenged pillar of the European alcohol policy discussion.

The central idea of Babor *et al.* is that all countries should adopt the authors' proposals presented as evidence-based alcohol policy. They write:

> With the growth of the knowledge base and the maturation of alcohol science, there is now a real opportunity to invest in evidence-based alcohol policies as an instrument of public health.[11]

The paternalistic/controlling strategies that the authors support are praised as 'cheap and effective', and consist of reducing the number of alcohol outlets as well as shortening their opening hours, greatly increasing taxes on alcohol, and punishing violations severely. All democratic–emancipatory strategy options that are in line with the *Ottawa Charter*, such as primary prevention, health education, health promotion and long-term treatment, are consistently rejected as 'expensive and ineffective.'

Despite the clear policy recommendations from Babor *et al.*, there is no reference to ethical questions. The implicit premise is that whatever measure for reducing alcohol consumption works, particularly if it creates no high extra costs for the government, must be adopted uncompromisingly. Questions such as whether the administration of a democratic society is allowed to paternalise, control and punish the vast majority of alcohol consumers who will never develop alcohol problems for the sake of a minority who will develop alcohol problems – in the words of Lloyd,[12] 'to punish many for the sins of a few' – were not addressed. Nor was there any reflection on the fact that a dramatic increase in alcohol prices has little impact on wealthy consumers, but dramatically affects the poorer sectors of society. As noted above, there is no mention in the summary that the empirical basis supporting the conclusions is far less conclusive than the reader of the summary might expect. However, the analysis of alcohol-related developments in Austria directly contradicts many conclusions of Babor *et al.*, as Uhl *et al.*[13,14] have quite clearly shown.

The effects of the 'alcopops' tax in Germany and the 'Pilate Fallacy'

Every researcher trained in statistics is aware that association must not be confused with causation, and that most data do not permit causal inference without making more or less plausible additional assumptions. To draw direct conclusions uncritically if the variables are concomitant is known as the 'Cum Hoc Fallacy',[2]* and if they are in successive order it is known as the 'Post Hoc Fallacy.'[2]† The problem for researchers is that they are permanently confronted with situations where their counterparts expect unconditional, simple, unequivocal and seemingly well-confirmed causal interpretations, which they cannot honestly produce. One approach for a scientist in this dilemma is to admit the problems openly, to formulate plausible assumptions explicitly, to argue these assumptions transparently (referring to existing research evidence, logic and plausibility), to interpret the available data based on these assumptions, and to admit ambiguities, uncertainties and other problems in the conclusions.

The other approach is to define the research questions and describe the plain results without interpretation. The researcher under such conditions can sit back and remain totally descriptive, knowing that the desired causal conclusions will be drawn by others without their having to 'get their hands dirty.' Setting up a situation in such a way that others inadvertently commit a fallacy – regardless of whether it is done on purpose or not – was termed a 'booby-trap' situation by Curtis:[2] 'a linguistic snare which is not itself fallacious, but may cause someone to inadvertently commit a fallacy.' If researchers are truly convinced that remaining descriptive is sufficient in a situation whenever they cannot make any sense out of their data, they are committing a serious fallacy themselves. By analogy with the biblical example of Pilate, who washed his hands of guilt after the trial of Christ, the term 'Pilate Fallacy' or 'Stay clean and have others commit the error you implicitly suggested Fallacy' is adequate. Staying strictly descriptive, and anticipating that the reader

---

* To be precise: 'Cum Hoc Ergo Propter Hoc Fallacy.'
† To be precise: 'Post Hoc Ergo Propter Hoc Fallacy.'

will commit all the logical fallacies necessary to arrive at the very conclusions that the scientist shares, is by no means scientific objectivity. If done unintentionally, it constitutes a form of ignorance, and if done intentionally it is a very subtle form of intent to mislead.

Scientific literature is full of examples of the 'Pilate Fallacy.' A good recent example is the evaluation of the new German 'alcopops'* law. Germany introduced a new specific alcopops tax and immediately after it was imposed, alcopops sales fell dramatically. Parallel with this, an almost identical decrease in alcopops sales occurred in Austria, where no such tax had been imposed. This suggests that the alcopops fashion had vanished independently or almost independently of any new taxes. The aims of the new tax were purely descriptive: 'The law aims at lower alcopops consumption through higher prices.' The German Federal Centre for Health Education[15] was also purely descriptive when reporting the results of an evaluation of its effects:

> Consumption of spirits-based alcopops as well as total alcohol consumption has moved in the intended direction . . . The consumption of spirits-based alcopops by 12- to 17-year-old youths declined significantly from 2004 through 2005 in frequency as well as quantity.

In other words, the authors never said explicitly that there was a causal relationship between the new tax and the reduction in sales, but they never called for caution when interpreting the results either, and there was not the slightest explicit hint that the association might be a mere coincidence. On the basis of this report, the German Ministry of Finance,[16] which had commissioned the study initially, interpreted it unconditionally and explicitly as showing that there was a causal relationship: 'The conclusion is that the introduction of the alcopops tax increased the price of spirits-based alcopops, which caused a considerable reduction in demand.' No one protested.

The conflict between industry and the public health sector and the 'Bifurcation Fallacy'

If parents are afraid that they may have a hard time convincing their small child to go to bed straight away, a popular trick is to ask 'Do you want to brush your teeth first and then put on your pyjamas, or do you want to do it the other way round?' This dupes the child into believing

* Alcopops are pre-mixed alcoholic beverages, usually marketed in small bottles of volume less than 250ml, with an average alcohol content somewhat above that of average beer. Because of their sweetness and trendy design they are criticised for appealing particularly to minors.

that there are only two options available, and also that he or she can freely decide what to do. If the parents are lucky, the child does not realise that the most attractive third option would be to stay up longer. To see only two options if there are actually more than two is termed the 'Bifurcation Fallacy.'[2] A similar strategy is currently being used by the advocates of a strict alcohol and tobacco control policy. They present the issue exclusively as a struggle between a very potent industry and an under-resourced public health sector, sometimes even demanding that research should unconditionally join the side of the public health sector in order to counterbalance some of the inequalities. This bipolar reductionism covers up the fact that there are more than two stake-holders involved in this conflict. Not considered to be partners in this discourse, for example, are consumers who perceive smoking cigarettes and/or drinking alcohol as an inalienable right, or workers involved in the production and trading of these commodities.

'Is cannabis dangerous?' and the 'Bifurcation Fallacy'

A standard question about cannabis is 'Is it harmless or dangerous?' Since this question is always asked in relation to cannabis policy options, the implicit ethical premise is that dangerous objects and activities must be forbidden. The flaw in this question is that a continuous quantitative scale of 'risk of adverse outcomes' is presented as a dichotomy – harmless versus dangerous. Such a dichotomy requires the definition of a precise cut-off point. To present it as a dichotomy is an example of the 'Bifurcation Fallacy' again.

It is a truism that hardly any behaviour is completely without risk. Some people suffocate while trying to drink a glass of water, others break their necks as they fall out of their beds, and many die while driving motor vehicles or climbing mountains. However, no one has ever considered outlawing the drinking of water, sleeping at night or driving motor vehicles, and only a few have demanded the outlawing of mountain climbing. Obviously the implicit simple ethical principle that everything dangerous must be forbidden has no chance of being accepted as a basic principle if it is made explicit and generalised. However, only a few individuals will object if they are confronted with such an implicit principle in areas where they are in favour of a strict control policy anyway. Logic is commonly welcome only if it serves to refute conclusions that one rejects emotionally, but little appreciated if it interferes with conclusions that one accepts emotionally.

Researchers at least should be able to get beyond this kind of subjectivism. Adequate research concerning the dangers associated with cannabis use or other activities should assess the different dimensions of risk and do so quantitatively. Adequate research should also compare the risk for a variety of different legal and illegal behaviours to compare them, and assess objective and subjective benefits to counterbalance these risks. The simple question 'Is cannabis dangerous?' is a perfect example of the fact that not only answers but also questions can be completely wrong.

Gateway theory and the 'Post Hoc Fallacy' and the 'Loaded Words Fallacy'

The gateway theory, which claims that cannabis consumption is associated with an elevated risk of subsequent heroin use, has been a highly popular argument in cannabis policy discussion for many decades. The theory has hardly ever been specified precisely enough to enable serious conclusions based on it to be drawn. The fact that most heroin users have used cannabis previously is interpreted by some as proving that cannabis consumption causally increases the risk of later heroin consumption – a classical 'Post Hoc Fallacy.'[2]* It is equally inadequate to reject the existence of a causal association between cannabis and heroin consumption by arguing that all heroin users have previously used not only cannabis but also milk, because the cannabis and heroin consumption correlates whereas the milk and heroin consumption does not.

It is very peculiar that supporting the gateway theory is virtually synonymous with rejecting a liberal cannabis policy, and that rejecting the gateway theory is synonymous with supporting such a policy. This is hard to understand logically, as the liberal Dutch cannabis policy is explicitly founded on accepting a gateway theory, explaining the relationship by a social factor. The Dutch policy was introduced in order to separate the cannabis market from the heroin market and so prevent cannabis users from running an elevated risk of coming into contact with heroin. Even if the relationship between cannabis and heroin consumption cannot be explained by social factors but only by individual ones, via an elevated susceptibility to drug use, this would not justify a strict cannabis policy either. If two substances serve a similar function and an intervention makes one of them less available, one would expect that the other substance would become more popular. Economic theory suggests that, if someone is fond of apples and pears, to make one of these fruits unavailable will very likely enhance their consumption of the other. It may well be, for instance, that the higher prevalence of cannabis use in

* The 'Post Hoc Ergo Propter Hoc Fallacy' refers to the assumption that because one thing follows another the one thing was caused by the other.

the USA is a result of making alcohol very difficult for youngsters to obtain.

Overall, the gateway theory is a very good example of two groups trying to get support for their favoured drug policy option by using the term 'gateway theory' primarily because of its connotation – what methodologists call the 'Loaded Words Fallacy'[2]* – even though the denotative content, if analysed logically, suggests exactly the opposite policy.

Alcohol consumption and traffic risk, and the 'Fallacy of Suppressed Evidence'

The most famous project on the relationship between alcohol consumption and traffic risk is the Grand Rapids Study by Borkenstein *et al.*[17] It was a well-designed, large roadside and case–control study, and served as the scientific basis for introducing specific blood alcohol concentration (BAC) limits in many European countries. When the data were analysed, the authors found an unexpected result. The risk of traffic accidents was half as high for drivers with a BAC around 0.02% as it was for drivers who were completely sober. The initial interpretation was that small amounts of alcohol enhance driving capability, and this phenomenon was named the 'Grand Rapids Dip.' When Hurst[18] reanalysed the data according to strata of drivers with similar alcohol consumption, he found that the risk of causing an accident while under the influence of alcohol increased constantly as the BAC levels increased, but he also found that abstainers and near-abstainers were more than four times as dangerous in a sober state as sober daily drinkers. Daily drinkers, according to this analysis, reached the level of risk that sober abstainers only had when they drank up to 0.1% – which is twice the level that a driver is allowed to reach in most European countries nowadays. Edwards *et al.*,[19] who wrote the predecessor to the previously mentioned book, *Alcohol, No Ordinary Commodity*, decided to describe only the first effect, namely that any amount of alcohol increases the risk of traffic accidents, and to withhold any mention of the second effect, namely that abstainers and near-abstainers in a sober state constituted a major traffic risk. In order to conceal the latter fact, they normed the risk level at 0% BAC as 1, and thereby concealed the story that they did not want to communicate – a classical 'Fallacy of Suppressed Evidence', which is hard to justify from a scientific point of view.[13]

---

* The 'Loaded Words Fallacy' refers to the deliberate use of prejudiced terms.

Economic costs of substance abuse and the 'Naive Fallacy'

Single *et al.*[20] have developed internationally accepted guidelines to enumerate and aggregate the economic costs of problematic substance use. Those costs have been estimated to represent between 2.7% and 5.0% of the gross national product (GNP).[21,22] These incredibly high costs are very popular advocacy tools for justifying substance-related expenditure by police, justice, prevention, therapy, research and any other stakeholders involved. It is therefore understandable that there is little motivation for experts to analyse critically the logic behind these numbers. A systematic analysis makes it quickly evident that the concept is loaded with major logical and conceptual flaws. It is inconsistent in perspective and target criteria, it enumerates sometimes entirely fictitious costs, and it argues in a circular manner. Just a few examples are listed below to illustrate this.

- Since policy costs* and costs directly caused by the problem are aggregated to one sum of economic costs, the strange fact arises that the costs of the problem increase continuously the more we invest in combating it. That way any irrelevant problem, if we fight it determinedly enough, will appear as a very expensive major problem – a highly irrational circular way of arguing.[23]
- Since life years lost are quantified by what an average person would have produced in one year, the economic loss of four abusers dying 20 years early is equivalent to one person not born due to contraception or to one young migrant not allowed to enter the country.[24] What is not considered is that a non-existing person does not produce, but at the same time does not consume either – producing a zero balance for third parties.
- The costs for substance-related treatment are added as a cost factor, but offsetting costs avoided by the problem is not considered. This ignores, for instance, the fact that a person dying prematurely from cirrhosis of the liver cannot possibly die from cancer, and will never need intensive support in old age.[24]
- Since costs are accumulated regardless of whether they are avoidable or not, in line with the logic of these economic cost calculations, the economic loss of not being immortal is infinite.[24]

I could easily continue with more specific details showing that what is presented as the economic cost of substance abuse is based on a 'Naive

---

* Policy costs are costs for policy measures to reduce the tangible and intangible costs caused by the problem.

Fallacy', the commonly used term for hopelessly inappropriate simplistic miscalculation. If assessed seriously, the substance abuse-related costs that third parties have to bear are only a small proportion of what published figures try to make us believe. Indeed in some instances, such as cigarette smoking, the overall balance may even be in favour of third parties. For instance, smokers usually work, pay taxes and make pension contributions, but on average die much earlier and do not consume their pensions or require social care in old age.[24]

Substance-related death and the 'Naive Fallacy'

It is common practice to estimate the number of people who die annually as a result of alcohol, nicotine, drugs and other problem issues, and the numbers commonly presented are impressively high. Hardly anyone seems to care what the term 'substance-related death' actually means. These figures can be used to convince audiences with details when opening conferences, or as advocacy tools to highlight the importance of certain policy measures. Although 'substance-related' does not mean 'causally related' but simply 'associated', most individuals will instantly interpret the term as causal, and furthermore assume that there is only one cause logically assignable to a specific death. Both of these ideas are flawed and render the concept inconclusive – the product of a 'Naive Fallacy' again.

It is apparent that there are many circumstances and behaviours that have an impact on the duration of a person's life. Some factors increase life expectancy and others decrease it. The relevant factors are innumerable, and most of them interact in a complex manner. To make the problem immediately visible, if someone dies earlier than average due to either taking very little exercise or over-exercising, can we sensibly call them a 'victim of suboptimal exercise'? If, on the other hand, someone lives longer due to taking optimal exercise, can they be classified as a 'beneficiary of optimal exercise'? Exercise or lack of exercise is certainly not the only behaviour that determines a lifespan. If we accept the classifications of 'victim of suboptimal exercise' or 'beneficiary of optimal exercise', how many minutes, hours or days must the effect be maintained for in order to justify such a classification? Even more tricky, imagine that someone, as a result of several adverse social and private circumstances, becomes depressive and is on the verge of committing suicide, but decides to self-medicate with alcohol and therefore survives for two more years until they finally put an end to their life. Can this person, whose death is clearly alcohol related but who lived two years longer due to alcohol use, justly be classified as a 'victim of alcohol', or is it more appropriate to label them a 'beneficiary of alcohol' instead? Does it make sense also to label them a 'victim of adverse social conditions', a 'victim of personal problems', a 'victim of depression', a 'victim of an inappropriate psychiatric system, not taking care of their depression in time' or a victim of numerous other adverse conditions that we could identify in their life? Is this person not also a beneficiary of all the lifetime-enhancing positive conditions in their life? I think it is quite obvious that it makes little sense to enumerate the number of substance-related deaths, and that it is inappropriate to interpret substance-related deaths as causally substance-attributable deaths and to classify every case of death for numerous reasons simultaneously. If we do the latter, we arrive at a total sum of many hundred per cent.

However, it does make sense to try to assess the average number of years lost due to a certain situation, or to assess the number of disability-adjusted or quality-adjusted years of life lost, so long as this is done correctly in methodological terms. It also makes some sense to count the number of victims who die immediately after certain events, such as car accidents, substance overdose, and so on, but it makes no sense to try to quantify the overall number of people who die due to alcohol, nicotine, illicit drugs, etc.[25]

Drug policy discussion and the 'Bifurcation Fallacy'

A common dichotomy in early drug policy discussion was coercive treatment versus imprisonment. Later, the dominant dichotomy was legalisation versus criminalisation, or decriminalisation versus criminal-isation. Due to the fact that more and more different policy options have been tried in different countries and that, in addition, a variety of harm reduction measures have become more and more established, the impact of these simple polarities has systematically vanished, at least among experts. In political and media discussions, this simple way of scoring by associating one's own ethical preferences with generally accepted strat-egies, and contrasting this with a rather extremely formulated alternative that the majority rejects, is still a reality. In the latter form, this line of reasoning resembles the 'Straw Man Fallacy',[2] in which a counterargu-ment is produced to refute a fake argument, thus adding credibility to one's own argument.

Conclusion

Putting the finger on methodological problems and fallacies is commonly not appreciated by researchers whenever the critical remarks directly target their work. On the other hand, many researchers enjoy hearing such 'theoretical things' if they are described comprehensibly, and if this does not impact seriously on their everyday work. Virtually everyone is fond of critical theory if it helps to challenge the positions of disliked conclusions.

It may be atypical to believe that it makes sense to apply the basic principles of logic and methodology to one's own work and similarly to the work of others. The role of a researcher involves challenging all existing theories destructively, including one's own convictions and pet theories, an approach that is absolutely contrary to the role of an advocate, who tries to assemble evidence systematically in order to prove their point, and who is more interested in effect – if necessary by deceiving people – than in enhancing knowledge.

Researchers should be ready to accept this more difficult task in their daily work, empowered by the conviction that only actively removing logical obstacles can enable us to truly advance, rather than pretending to be moving them to our customers and often to ourselves.

References

1 Deschner KH. *Mörder Machen Geschichte [Murderers Make History]*. Basel: Lenos; 2003.
2 Curtis GN. The fallacy files; www.fallacyfiles.org/index.html (accessed 31 January 2006).
3 Hume DA. *A Treatise on Human Nature. Book 3 of Morals, Part I, of Virtue and Vice in General*; 1740. In: Watkins F (ed) *Theory of Politics*. Edinburgh: Nelson and Sons; 1951.
4 Moore GE. *Principia Ethica*. Cambridge: Cambridge University Press; 1903 (second paperback edition, 1960).
5 Uhl A. The limits of evaluation. In: Neaman R, Nilson M, Solberg U, editors. *Evaluation: a key tool for improving drug prevention*. EMCDDA Scientific Monograph Series No. 5. Lisbon: European Monitoring Centre for Drugs and Drug Addiction (EMCDDA); 2000.
6 Sackett DL, Rosenberg WMC, Gray M *et al*. Evidence-based medicine: what it is and what it isn't (editorial). *BMJ*. 1996; **312**: 71–2.
7 Hartnoll R. *Drugs and drug dependence: linking research, policy and practice background*. Paper presented to the Pompidou Group's Strategic Conference on Connecting Research, Policy and Practice, 6–7 April 2004. Strasbourg: Council of Europe Publishing; 2004.
8 Pirie M. *The Book of the Fallacy*. London: Routledge & Kegan Paul; 1985.
9 Pittman DJ, editor. *Alcoholism*. New York: Harper & Row; 1967.
10 World Health Organization. *Ottawa Charter*. Geneva: World Health Organization; 1986.
11 Babor TF, Caetano R, Casswell S *et al*. *Alcohol, No Ordinary Commodity. Research and public policy*. New York: Oxford University Press; 2003.
12 Lloyd PJ. The economics of regulation of alcohol distribution and consumption in Victoria. *Aust Econ Rev*. 1985; **12**: 16–29.
13 Uhl A, Beiglböck W, Fischer F *et al*. Alkoholpolitik in Österreich: status quo und perspektiven [Alcohol policy in Austria: status quo and perspectives]. In: Babor T, Caetano R, Casswell S *et al*., editors. *Alkohol: Kein gewöhnliches Konsumgut. Forschung und Alkoholpolitik [Alcohol: No ordinary commodity]*. Göttingen: Hogrefe; 2005.

14 Uhl A. *Alkoholpolitik und wissenschaftliche Forschung [Alcohol policy and scientific research].* Aufsatz zum Vortrag 'Wirksamkeit struktureller Prävention' bei der DHS Fachkonferenz 'Suchtprävention' ['Effectiveness of structural prevention' to the Symposium 'Prevention of Addiction' of the German Centre on Addiction problems], 8–10 November 2004, Bielefeld. Vienna: Ludwig-Boltzmann-Institut für Suchtforschung; 2005.

15 BZgA. *Entwicklung des Alkoholkonsums bei Jugendlichen unter besonderer Berücksichtigung der Konsumgewohnheiten von Alkopops [Trends in Alcohol Consumption in Young People, in Particular the Consumption of Alcopops].* Cologne: BZgA; 2005.

16 BMF. *Bericht der Bundesregierung über die Auswirkungen des Alkopopsteuergesetzes auf den Alkoholkonsum von Jugendlichen unter 18 Jahren sowie die Marktentwicklung von Alkopops und vergleichbaren Getränken [Report of the Federal Government on the Impact of the Alcopops Law on the Alcohol Consumption of Young People Below 18 Years of Age and Market Developments Concerning Alcopops and Comparable Beverages].* Berlin: Bundesministerium der Finanzen; 2005.

17 Borkenstein RF, Crowther RF, Shumate RP *et al. The Role of the Drinking Driver in Traffic Accidents.* Indianapolis, IN: Department of Police Administration, Indiana University; 1964 (reprinted in *Blutalkohol.* 1974; **11:** 1–131).

18 Hurst PM. Epidemiological aspects of alcohol in driver crashes and citations. *J Safety Res.* 1973; **5:** 130–47.

19 Edwards G, Anderson P, Babor TF *et al. Alcohol Policy and the Public Good.* Oxford: Oxford University Press; 1994.

20 Single E, Robson L, Easton B *et al. International Guidelines for Estimating the Costs of Substance Abuse. Summary of 2001 edition.* Ottowa: Canadian Centre on Substance Abuse; 2001.

21 Single E, Robson L, Xie X *et al. The Costs of Substance Abuse in Canada.* Ottawa: Canadian Centre on Substance Abuse; 1997.

22 Collins D, Lapsley H. *The Social Costs of Drug Abuse in Australia in 1988 and 1992.* National Drug Strategy Monograph Series, No. 30. Canberra: Australian Government Publishing Service; 1996.

23 Wagstaff A. Government prevention policy and the relevance of social cost estimates. *Br J Addiction.* 1987; **82:** 461–7.

24 Uhl A. Darstellung und kritische Analyse von Kostenberechnungen im Bereich des Substanzmissbrauchs [Description and critical analysis of cost calculations in the field of substance abuse]. *Sucht.* 2006; **52:** 121–32.

25 Uhl A. Todesfälle durch Substanzkonsum. Wie sinnvoll ist dieses Konzept? [Substance-related death. How sensible is this concept?] *Wien Z Suchtforsch.* 2002; **25:** 23–32.

Index